Mending Nerves

An Empathetic Journey with Multiple Sclerosis

ROBERT CUSINATO

◆ FriesenPress

Suite 300 - 990 Fort St
Victoria, BC, V8V 3K2
Canada

www.friesenpress.com

ISBN
978-1-03-910001-5 (Hardcover)
978-1-03-910000-8 (Paperback)
978-1-03-910002-2 (eBook)

1. BIOGRAPHY & AUTOBIOGRAPHY, MEDICAL

Distributed to the trade by The Ingram Book Company

Dedicated to those champions who carry the burden of multiple sclerosis and the zealous who propel them.

Thanks for your support! Enjoy Life!

Rob

Foreword

There are times in your life when your path has many possibilities and times when there are only a few options. It is what we do with those choices—how we forge ahead into unknown territory—that defines us. Ronald Reagan once said, "The future doesn't belong to the fainthearted. It belongs to the brave." He stated this after the Challenger disaster. Life is a challenge and we must be brave moving forward.

I met Rob Cusinato in my first year of university. Since then we have shared many memories and made our own forays into the unknowns of life. Rob and I have always had a great love for music. During the time Rob was writing this book, reminiscing about our friendship invoked in me the memory of a song called "Intelligent People" from the former lead singer of one of my favourite bands, Catherine Wheel. The song relays the message of a parent telling their child, "You've just gotta smile and hang out with intelligent people." To be with Rob and those we surrounded ourselves with in those formative years made me realize just how intelligent Rob is. Our friends helped support us in our goals, a true sign of intelligence.

Especially when it was tempting to sabotage a fellow student vying for the same spots in professional schools.

Rob is primarily responsible for the fact that I am a part of the great profession of physical therapy. His intelligence and foresight led him to suggest the field to me. In doing so, Rob changed my life. He provided me with a new path. You don't realize who is responsible for providing you with life-changing opportunities until you are older. I have never truly thanked him for showing me the path to my future, when I was twenty-one. Physical therapy has been good to me; I love my work.

I have witnessed Rob change the life of many patients. He continues to show his friends, family, and patients' new paths. I hope this book helps you find hope or a new path. Or perhaps it will simply make you run, dance, jump, squat, or take the stairs, because you can. We shouldn't take these things for granted, so stay active!

Multiple sclerosis (MS) is a disease affecting many people. Canada still has the highest rates per capita. It affects not only the afflicted person but alters the home and world in which they live. It changes family dynamics. My mother was diagnosed with MS in 2008. It has stripped her of her independence, left her in chronic pain, and changed my family forever.

Rob's book is designed to open our eyes as therapists, health-care workers, and people to the internal and external struggle for independence that those affected by MS endure. His words are a reminder to the health care professional that sympathy is not what a patient needs; we all must demonstrate empathy and understanding. They are a reminder of how, as therapists, we can help or harm our patients with the power of our words and non-verbal communication. His words are an eloquent and poignant reminder to healthcare professionals why we chose to do what we do.

To those who have MS, Rob will remind you that life is full of wonder, you must set goals, you are not alone, and it is alright to ask for help.

Ultimately, his book illustrates how one man manages to accept the change in his path and continues to change others. It is a reminder to all of us to be empathetic and not to be afraid to have difficult conversations with our friends and family.

I implore each of you to donate to MS charities and to support research. Research is going to change lives!

Thank you, Rob, for this insightful book.

Ryan Thomas

TODAY

An Imperfect Beginning to a Perfect Day

BEEP! BEEP! BEEP! BEEP! BEEP!

"Already? Did I even fall asleep? What day is it anyways? I think it's Tuesday. I need to get up and get ready for work. Maybe I'll just call in. Nope. I better get up."

The incessant squawking of his phone beckoned. It was six o'clock in the morning. Lobio was momentarily startled, and realized that as he was unnerved, the control of his extremities was compromised considerably more than it routinely was. Reaching to disable the alarm, his first attempt was unsuccessful. His index finger struck everything except the "Stop" icon. He hoped that the clamour would not awaken the rest of the family. They had likely acclimated to his rituals. His intention tremor was characterized by abnormal movement, incoordination, and shaking when he moved the affected body part voluntarily. The diminished control of his right hand demonstrated that, today, just like last night when he fell asleep, he had multiple sclerosis (MS). Lobio fantasized that one night he might sleep it off.

To be candid, an intense urgency from deep within his nether regions would ordinarily awaken him before the alarm hollered. In this instance the silence was deafening; PEE! PEE! PEE! "The bathroom is so close but so far away," Lobio mused.

The dilemma was that he could not move fast, especially in the morning. Upon awakening, his legs were especially tight, and they were weighted down by muscle spasticity, neuropathic burning, and numbness. The spasticity presented as stiffness and tightness in his muscles, especially in his lower extremities. Normal, smooth movement would be restricted. "Neuropathic" implied damage to nerves resulting in impaired sensation over the area of the nerve's distribution. Lobio sat on the side of the bed and gained his composure. "Deep breath. Here we go. Time to get up and start the day."

He was transitioning from sitting to standing better these days because he had been working on it. Once standing, he could not just walk away. It was time for his legs to get the shake out of them, just like his arms did when he reached out toward the phone. He steadied himself with his hand on the wall and did "the dance." The cadence of his shaking remained consistent, but the amplitude gradually faded until after about ten seconds he was relatively still. He likened this to his nervous system rebooting.

His gait was characterized by a wide base of support with short and shaky steps. He was somewhat peg-legged as the spasticity restricted his knees from effectively bending, especially his right. The furniture and walls did not need to speak as they provided him with support and encouragement during the initial trek. Without this tacit accord his trip to the bathroom would be even more perilous. The walls were emblazoned with his oily fingerprints, only to remind him further that they had forged a kinship.

Lobio would make it to the bathroom eventually. Standing to urinate was a distant memory. Sitting down at the toilet was now commonplace. In fact, the thought of entering a public restroom where the stalls were occupied and only a urinal was available was daunting. Most of the time it was not because of "number two" that he needed a stall. The resolution to sit down on the toilet was based on self-analysis. Two factors came into play. One, his standing balance, whether static or dynamic, was subpar. "Static" refers to balance while the base of support remains still, while "dynamic" implies balance with movement of the support base. He was certainly a fall risk. The last thing that Lobio needed was a laceration, a fracture, or even worse, a head injury. The other factor in his decision to sit was that it could take him as long as five minutes to urinate. His bladder dysfunction was "neurogenic," meaning that his bladder control issues were the result of damage to his nervous system. There was more stopping and going than the traffic of a busy downtown metropolis. Often, some coaxing with his fingers jabbed deeply into his lower abdomen could force out a little more flow. Eventually he was rewarded with relief.

After using the washroom in the morning, Lobio would move on to his next task. He would consume a couple large glasses of water. This was timed strategically so that he could relieve himself just before he left for work, in about two hours. He would not drink anything else until he was at work. His bladder never fully emptied and if urgency struck him while he was driving, the consequences could be disastrous. This was a chance that he had learned not to take. Along with his water he would take his morning medication and a small assortment of vitamins.

Next, a prolonged warm shower provided him with benefits that extended far beyond cleansing his body. It awakened him and prepared him for the day that lay ahead. He also focused on his cognition and speech while the warm water spattered his body. He challenged his memory by recalling the events of recent and distant history. He would cogitate on math problems, inspired by his daughter's schoolwork. The intention tremor that thwarted him was not isolated to his arms and legs. This dysfunction also afflicted his tongue and jaw. The result was a speech hardship that only he noticed, at least at that point. There were words that gave him difficulty. He would quietly enunciate these words as he showered. "Specifically. Pressure. Exercise. Probably. Firefighter. Sclerosis."

The greatest benefit offered by a shower was that it reduced the spasticity in his legs. His muscles became supple and his joints moved more freely. In fact, aside from ataxia (an uncoordinated feeling of drunkenness), his gait pattern was almost normal. After the warm shower he could bend his knees with greater fluidity. He would still rely on the walls for support but not for every step. He felt free. Alas, it was time for him to dry off, put on deodorant, apply lotion, get dressed, and shave; all while sitting down.

He proceeded to the kitchen. Breakfast most often included fruit, cereal, toast with almond butter, and a hard-boiled egg. He would fight the urge to drink anything more. In fact, he would often eat his cereal dry, keeping away from more liquid. "I already drank a large volume of water. I better not drink any more. Not yet anyways," he would think.

It was now time to ensure that the kids were ready for school. Christine, Lobio's wife, had already left for work.

After breakfast, he was generally granted the luxury of a little free time to exercise while he read or listened to music. Sit-ups, planks, squats, and stretches comprised his morning exercise regimen. His song choices and playlists were reflective of his mood that day. No matter what he chose, music was a delight to more than just his ears. The lyrics comforted him as they helped him deal with his reality. There was always a different message conveyed. The theme of each song varied. It might be love or hate. Triumph or tragedy. Success or failure. However, no matter the theme, every song reminded him of the same four words: "I AM NOT ALONE!"

Then it would be time for him to brush his teeth and don his coat and shoes, once again all sitting down. Most of his world was spent methodically on his butt and not on his feet. Time to ensure that the kids caught their respective buses and then he could head to work. Each morning he hoped there would be no delays on the way to work because when he finally arrived, it would be time to relieve himself again.

The drive was sometimes eventful. He made decisions that he felt were in his own best interest, and the interest of those driving around him. First and foremost, he kept his distance. He would not tail anyone. He knew that both his reaction time and the control of his right leg were not as quick as most and he took that into consideration when he was behind the wheel. He maintained significant space between his vehicle and the one in front. He was not heavy on the gas pedal. When he was approaching a stop, especially if traffic was heavy, his right hand grasped the emergency brake. He was never forced to engage this device, but it gave him peace of mind knowing that he could if needed. As he did his due diligence, it did not stop others from zipping by, laying on their horns, or providing hand gestures that needed no interpretation.

"That's nice. If only you knew. Maybe you would understand. What's your rush anyways? Is somebody chasing you?"

Lobio recently asked Christine, "Have they changed the driving laws? Not many seem to signal anymore. It used to be just the odd driver. Now it seems that so many don't."

"I have noticed that too", she agreed.

Perhaps for many it was not a big deal, but it was to Lobio. Because his reaction times were not as quick as they used to be, he was much more confident behind the wheel when there was a significant amount of space between his vehicle and the one ahead. However, when he left adequate space, drivers would inevitably squeeze in ahead of him, often without signaling. He was vigilant about the vehicles around him, but when they failed to signal, Lobio could not anticipate their respective moves. He was sure there were others around like him and didn't think it was too much to ask to signal. Driving was a privilege.

When he arrived at work, the first thing he needed to do was get to the washroom. Round two on the toilet. Relief . . . again.

At around 8:25 a.m., he could be found sitting in the staff room getting ready for his workday. At half past eight a second alarm would go off. It was time to work. If he slept relatively well it would just be a tough day. If he didn't sleep well it would be a genuinely tough day. It only took two and a half hours from the time that he woke up to get to that point. It was now routine for him.

Lobio was a physiotherapist. In fact, he was a physiotherapist long before he carried the burden of MS. He ended up in a career that could not be more suited to the person he was. He worked primarily in the outpatient department within a local hospital. Ironically, most clients that he treated were suffering from a variety of neurological impairments, including MS. He grabbed his files for the day and his water bottle, all with his left. His right hand and arm were reserved for his forearm crutch and that alone. Who and what was awaiting him on the other side of the door? "Stand up. Stabilize. Deep breath. In through the nose and out through the mouth. I can do this (usually). Walk. Open the door . . ."

YESTERDAY

Fantasizing with Open Eyes

As the distant stars opened their eyes, the brilliant moon was already awake and alert. It was staring acutely through the gap between the curtains. A faint illumination permeated the darkened bedroom. The songs of chirping crickets filled Lobio's ears. Despite the late hour, his eyes were wide open. As he lay on his back, he gazed upward, remaining completely still. His thoughts were racing. It was one of those evenings when drifting off seemed hopeless. He was envisioning his future life plastered on the ceiling above. His body reminded him that it was time to sleep but his mind had other ideas. It had been a memorable day. Earlier, he had graduated with a Bachelor of Science in biology from the local university. This was a tremendous achievement for him, and it was one he would never undervalue—but now what? Where would he go from here? He was only twenty-two years old and there was still so much to learn. He recalled his final year of high school when he participated in the co-op program and was placed in a local hospital. He had expressed an interest in the medical field. While at the hospital, he spent a month in the physiotherapy department. This was an eye-opening experience. Before that placement, Lobio was not even aware of physiotherapy. "One day you will be a physiotherapist," his supervisor declared. The seed was planted and when the right time came, he applied. He knew what he wanted but it was not in his hands. He waited.

"Lobio, you've got mail." The weathered, middle-aged man laboured downstairs, holding a stamped envelope in his roughened hand. With the other, he steadied a cup of espresso that was fragranced with grappa. Hanging on for dear life in the corner of his mouth was a smouldering cigarette. There was always something very comforting about the mingled aroma of cigarette smoke, grappa, and coffee. Like the ethereal caress of a mother's delicate hand on the face of her child, it reminded Lobio that he was home! The man's body was muscular and chiseled, but it was also overlaid with scrapes, bruises, and scars. Years of hard work in construction had left their mark. On his head was a ratty, old, oversized baseball cap that he must have plucked from the depths of the entrance closet. The front was adorned with the logo of a minor league baseball team from Central America. The man could care less as long as the cap had a visor that would shield the sun from his eyes. He was also wearing a damaged pair of glasses that he probably discovered on the street. The lenses were scratched. In fact, there were times when one of the lenses was missing altogether. Perhaps they helped him to see better but Lobio believed that they were just a placebo. The man was preparing to head out for another arduous day of work during which he would lay tile for a fortunate homeowner. He was Lobio's father. It was he who had nicknamed his eldest son "Lobio" and that name stuck.

It was the early summer of 1994. The exact date escaped Lobio. This was unusual because he was told by many that his memory, especially regarding dates of events, was unparalleled. He recalled that it was the beginning of summer vacation. School was out. It was a pleasing day and he was indolently nestled on the basement couch, still snug in his pajamas. He was watching a movie on TV with his brothers. Jaws 2 to be exact. They watched the film as they waited for a soccer game to come on. The FIFA World Cup was taking place in the United States and Lobio's beloved Italy would soon be battling powerhouse Brazil in the final, but not that day. Lobio was Canadian by birth, Italian by blood, and very proud of both.

The letter he was holding was from one of the universities he had applied to. He knew immediately what this was. He was instantly filled with emotion. He felt anxiety stir deep within his viscera. It wasn't the spine-tingling scene in the movie that was making him feel this way. It was the mysterious contents of the letter. With great trepidation he tore open the envelope. He wished he could remember the exact words. He only had to read the first few. "Elation" was the best word to describe the emotion that filled him. He had been accepted into the school of physical therapy. He immediately knew that his career path was laid out in front of him. With diligent study habits, he would become a physiotherapist and after three years of school, he would begin the next chapter of his life—a chapter that would presumably encompass the next few decades. Maybe more.

His father had not yet left for work. He was the first one that Lobio shared this monumental news with. As a hard-working construction worker, he was more than happy that Lobio would not have to endure the same "battles" that he had to in his career. Lobio's supple hands were destined for therapeutic human touch, not cement. Lobio subsequently shared this news with his three younger brothers who were also home. He hoped they were happy, but he knew that they were more concerned with the weather outside, and rightfully so. A beautiful, clear summer day provided an invitation for many a game. Kevin, the second oldest, was triumphant as he would finally have a bedroom to himself. Trying to fall asleep with a roommate that sounded like a classic muscle car with a faulty muffler was one of the most challenging tasks of Lobio's daily routine. He loved his brother so much but.... "Shut up already!"

Lobio kept a hockey stick at his bedside so he could jab Kevin in the ribs and settle his breathing when needed.

His mother was already at work where she was employed as a teacher, yet he had no hesitation about disturbing her while she taught. He was thrilled to share the news of his acceptance with her, so he made the call. Remember those days when we used our land lines to make phone calls? There was something nostalgic about hearing a voice on the other end of a line from a phone that was attached to the wall by a coiled cord. He could sense her joy on the other end, and her ear-to-ear grin. He could also hear relief in her voice as she must have thought: "One down. Three to go!"

Lobio had no hesitation about accepting a seat in this program. In about three short months he would be moving away from home and living on his own. This was another step in the metamorphosis into manhood.

"Freedom! To save some money, I will have pasta for breakfast, lunch, and dinner for the next few years. Occasionally I will treat myself to some gourmet mac and cheese."

September 1994: his first day at a distant university, studying physical therapy. Lobio was thrust, by choice, into a classroom with several other lost comrades. The nervousness and enthusiasm were palpable. His thoughts were scattered: "Where should I sit? What profound narrative will come from the mouth of my first lecturer? Did I lock the front door? Is the stove turned off? Crap. I hope that I covered all the bases. What shape of pasta noodle am I going to eat tonight? What am I going to wear tomorrow? What floor in my apartment building is the laundry room on? Stop. Focus. Listen. Learn."

This was the first time he was away from the familiarity of home. He was at school in a city two hours from the comfort of the family home. In addition to his comprehensive studies, he would have to cook for himself, do his own laundry, scrub down the bathroom (maybe), keep up on his bills, pay rent, walk a couple kilometers to school, and keep his bachelor apartment clean and tidy; the latter just in case his mother visited. These were responsibilities that he took for granted. In fact, like many others, he would put things off until the next day or the day after that. Little did he know that these tedious, monotonous, and ubiquitous tasks would become responsibilities that he would crave in the future.

Lobio was in a class of sixty-four: one of the fewer than 10 percent applying to this university who had been offered a seat in the program. There were two familiar faces. One of these, George, became a cherished friend, and one of Lobio's roommates. When George went home for the weekend, he would not return empty-handed. The freezer would inevitably be packed with mouth-watering Greek food prepared by his mother. Before Lobio and his two other roommates even had a chance, George would often devour everything within the first few days, leaving the others with piles of empty plates and plastic containers on the kitchen counter and the coffee table. That's okay because the roommates got him back when they moved all his belongings, including his bedroom furniture, into the kitchen one evening when he was out. But it didn't faze him. When they proceeded to prepare breakfast the following morning, George was sound asleep on his bed in the middle of the kitchen. The others couldn't get to the fridge. Once again, George had the last laugh.

Another classmate had also become a friend and eventually a co-worker of Lobio's. All his other classmates were strangers to him. It was a diverse group representing individuals from different cities and backgrounds. They became a classroom of equals who encouraged and supported each other. Not only did they get to know each other's personalities, but they also became familiar with each other's bodies. They had to for the sake of learning! The study of physical therapy was not necessarily difficult, but it was assuredly a great deal of work. The students spent a significant amount of time in the classroom, learning theory, as well as in the lab, practicing hands-on techniques.

There were three main subsections of physical therapy that the curriculum focused on. They studied physical therapy as it applied to individuals suffering from musculoskeletal disorders, neurological disorders, and cardiorespiratory disorders.

Like the public, the students were most familiar with physical therapy aimed at treating musculoskeletal disorders. Ankle sprain. "Pulled" hamstring. Shoulder dislocation. Rotator cuff tear. Carpal tunnel syndrome. Broken hip. Sciatica. Low back strain. Whiplash. Knee replacement. The list went on and on. This was a small set of diagnoses for which an individual might seek the help of a physiotherapist. The neurological and cardiorespiratory subsections were less familiar and likely less understood by not only future physiotherapists but by everyone in general. To be honest, Lobio knew very little about the role that physical therapy played in the rehabilitation of these conditions. In his studies, he would soon find out what a significant difference a physiotherapist could make.

There were a vast number of conditions that encompassed the cardiorespiratory subsection. There were conditions such as myocardial infarction (heart attack), congestive heart failure, chronic obstructive pulmonary disease, emphysema, asthma, pulmonary fibrosis, cystic fibrosis, and interstitial lung disease. There were also individuals who had undergone cardiac surgery, thoracic surgery, or lung transplantation who would require post-operative rehabilitation. Deep breathing, coughing, strengthening, and conditioning exercises would be advised. Occasionally hands-on techniques such as chest percussion were incorporated. A well-trained physiotherapist would know when and how to progress an individual.

There were also several conditions that comprised the neurological subsection. There were individuals suffering from a cerebrovascular accident (commonly referred to as a "stroke"). There were those suffering from a traumatic brain injury. There were those suffering from a spinal cord injury. There were others afflicted by a neuromuscular disease, such as Lou Gehrig's disease (ALS), Parkinson's disease, or MS; the latter Lobio would eventually become all too familiar with. These represent a myriad of conditions affecting the nervous system, that could impair an individual's ability to eat, swallow, speak, see, smell, hear, feel, sleep, balance, and walk. Bowel dysfunction, bladder dysfunction, or both are unfortunately common. Incoordination and a lack of control of an individual's head, trunk, arms, or legs is also not uncommon. Range of motion, strengthening, conditioning, balance, coordination, and walking exercises are advised. Hands-on techniques that facilitate and guide the individual are used to help them regain control and normalize movement as much as possible. Education regarding the use of a walking aid or other assistive device is also very important. A well-trained physiotherapist would be equipped with knowledge and a repertoire of tools to aid the client in achieving their realistic goals.

Lobio attended physical therapy school between 1994 and 1997. In that relatively short period of time, he was bombarded with a significant amount of information. There was so much to learn and in so little time. He learned what the body looked like both on the outside and on the inside and how several of the "ticking parts" functioned. He was enlightened as to what could happen to various parts of the body when "things went wrong." Most importantly, he appreciated what he could do, as a future physiotherapist, to help an individual deal with those issues from a physical standpoint. Lobio understood that specific neurological lesions, no matter the diagnosis, often demonstrated similar clinical signs and symptoms. Damage to one side of the brain caused by any of the diagnoses could cause impairments to the other side of the body, such as a loss of range of motion, weakness, incoordination, or spasticity. Damage to parts of the left brain could cause impairments of speech. Aphasia, the inability to understand or express speech, could occur. Swallowing difficulties could be encountered.

Lobio recalled his introduction to clinical expressive (Broca's) aphasia. This type of aphasia was characterized by a difficulty producing language while comprehension remained intact. He met an elderly male, Chuck, who resided in a long-term care facility. Chuck had suffered a left-sided stroke and his speech was severely impaired. Lobio was advised by his co-workers that Chuck's responses would be indecipherable. Lobio still initiated some small talk to establish a rapport.

"Hi. I'm Lobio and I will be your physiotherapist. It's a pleasure to meet you. What is your name?"

Chuck's response, "Do-do-do-do."

"How old are you?"

"Do-do-do-do."

"How long have you lived at this residence?"

"Do-do-do-do."

"How is the food here?"

"Shit."

Chuck giggled. So did Lobio. He soon discovered that in addition to "do-do-do-do" and "shit," Chuck could say "buck off."

Lobio felt that it must be terrible to suffer from an inability to express oneself. Trapped. Knowing what you wanted but unable to convey that message and often settling for nothing but frustration. "Poor Chuck. I guess that the middle finger will just have to do. I think that it means, 'get lost.' Maybe it means, 'I need something but I'm tired of trying to explain what it is that I need so I give up.' He is surrounded by so many people, yet he is so alone."

Damage to the right side of the brain could impair intuitive thinking and spatial recognition, the ability to understand the relationship between objects in space. Individuals with right-sided brain lesions, especially over the frontal lobe, could exhibit impulsive behaviours. Damage to the cerebellum could result in impairments with respect to coordination, motor control, stability and, balance. Therefore, walking abilities on level surfaces, uneven surfaces, or stairs could be and often were affected. Reflex changes were also characteristic, either exaggerated or absent, depending on the part of the nervous system that was damaged.

So, what did Lobio learn about MS? Not much. This was neither a knock to the school nor the education he received. He could honestly say that he owed so much to this education and his subsequent employment as a physiotherapist. What he did learn during the program was that there were four types of MS. Relapsing-remitting MS demonstrates a brief period of one or more flare-ups, with new symptoms appearing, sometimes with complete recovery; this is the most common type of MS. Secondary-progressive MS demonstrates a gradual worsening of symptoms over time, with the presence or absence of flare-ups. Primary-progressive MS demonstrates a gradual worsening of symptoms with no flare-ups. Progressive-relapsing MS is the rarest type and demonstrates a gradual worsening of symptoms with occasional flare-ups not followed by recovery. Lobio learned that MS was a disease of the central nervous system and that the physical impairments varied depending on which part of the brain, spinal cord, or both demonstrated lesions. He learned that individuals with MS could be sensitive to heat. This meant that they should avoid hot weather, hot showers, baths, and overexerting themselves. He would find out firsthand that this was a vast understatement, at least for him. It was sensitivity to heat that made Lobio begin to suspect he might have MS.

June 1997. Once again, the exact day escaped Lobio. He had just graduated from the school of physical therapy. Leading up to his graduation, he had job interviews with a few local facilities. There was no shortage of work for a new physical therapy graduate.

At the age of twenty-five, Lobio began his career as a physiotherapist. He was hired by a local hospital. On his first day of work, he was certainly overdressed. Any more formal, and one would have thought he was going to a wedding. Though he was offered many job opportunities through the years, he remained employed at the hospital. He worked in multiple departments and with a varied clientele—individuals of all ages afflicted with musculoskeletal, cardiorespiratory, and/or neurological impairments. More recently, he split his time between the outpatient department and the pulmonary rehabilitation program.

Despite his training, most of his education came from working with his clients. What he learned from them was so vast in comparison to what he had learned in school. Any healthcare professional would attest to the same. Through his work with clients, he became aware of the pathophysiology (disease process) of so many health conditions. Eventually this education would serve him well as he sought answers when confronted with his own health dilemma.

Ascending with
Minor Turbulence

Lobio's life could not have been brighter. His employment as a physiotherapist provided him with a great sense of fulfillment as well as a steady source of income. He was excited that he was in a profession that was not only in high demand, but was also deeply gratifying, as he knew he was serving others. There were so many opportunities. And not many people could say that they went to work in jogging pants while serving so many fun and interesting people all the while being well-compensated.

For the next decade, life was routine, but it could also be described as fun and full of happiness. Lobio got married; became a father; purchased his first home; enjoyed concerts, live sporting events, and movies; and attended many social gatherings without giving them a second thought. Soccer continued to be a staple interest. It provided him with a regular activity to look forward to. He would often reflect on how this sport entered his life. When Lobio was five, his mother registered him to play in a T-ball league. At the time, he was very shy and reserved. She wanted to introduce him to an activity in which he battled with teammates who shared a common goal. As it turned out, he enjoyed picking dandelions in the outfield more, while his oversized yellow baseball cap covered his ears. When he did pay attention and ran to make a play, apparently, he was not fast enough.

"You run like you have a piano on your back," one of his coaches hollered as he was running the bases.

"I might run faster if you dangle a dandelion in front of me," Lobio thought to himself.

He recalled that when he was up to bat, the outfielders from the opposition would push in close to the infield. He was credited with one home run in two years and it was not the result of a skillful, high-powered hit. It was the culmination of multiple errors by the opposing team as Lobio rounded the bases. It was exciting for a few minutes but in the end, it did not matter to Lobio that much. Baseball was a beautiful sport in which the strategies required to win were fascinating. However, baseball was never meant for him, at least not at a competitive level.

When Lobio was in first grade, a classmate introduced him to a simple game in which the players would chase a ball around and strike it with their feet. They could never touch the ball with their hands and the aim was to kick the ball into the opponent's goal. Lobio found his sport and he never looked back. It was surprising that being of Italian heritage, he did not actually find it sooner. Lobio also found his speed.

"I guess the piano fell off my back."

When he met Christine over a quarter of a century ago, she soon learned of his passion for soccer. As much as he loved her, she came to know that soccer was his first love. A long time ago she inquired, "Are you ever going to stop playing soccer?"

Lobio's response was blunt: "When my legs fall off!"

His legs never did fall off. However, having legs while eventually not being able to use them for soccer would ignite many negative feelings. He competed in the sport for nearly four decades.

When the time came, it was a very difficult breakup. Dealing with this loss and the emotions that came with it was the starting point of his new life.

The year 2005 was one of the most memorable of Lobio's life for a couple of reasons. It was both the toughest and the happiest year. Firstly, his father suffered an untimely death on March 8. His short, progressive illness tested Lobio's emotional stability. When death came, it was both gut-wrenching and a relief, as his father had suffered horribly during the preceding four months. Prior to his father's illness, Lobio had been cultivating a relationship with him that extended beyond father and son; they were becoming close friends.

The week following his father's death, Lobio and Christine received a much-anticipated phone call from an adoption agency. On March 17 to be exact. A little girl from China matched their profile and had been selected for them to adopt. Lobio's father, who was so excited about being a grandfather for the first time, missed this phone call by just over a week. He was laid to rest eternally on March 11. Reviewing their daughter's paperwork revealed that she was chosen for them on March 11, which also happened to be Lobio's thirty-third birthday. Lili was born in China and introduced to Lobio and Christine at ten months. She was a priceless gift.

In hindsight, 2010 was also one of the greatest years of Lobio's life; that year, he and Christine adopted another child. Lili chose a name for him: Andrew. He was from South Korea, and was an active child, full of energy and full of life. He was also a priceless gift to their family. There was never a shortage of laughs with this little guy. He wanted to run, play soccer, go to the park, ride his bike, swim, play with his toys, read comic books, play the drums, or play video games. And Lobio knew that Andrew deserved it. "A union with the Far East gave birth to a family," he thought.

Lobio had more than he could have ever wanted: health, happiness, freedom, steady and rewarding employment, the desire and ability to travel, soccer, a beautiful family, and so many wonderful people surrounding him. However, one of the certainties in life is that it is filled with uncertainties.

Things were about to change.

A Redundant Knock
on the Door

What were the symptoms that ultimately led to Lobio's diagnosis? How did he arrive here? He was frequently asked this. He was asked by those closest to him and he was often asked by his clients. He told them the truth.

"Raisins. That's what did it. Even the sight of one of those vile little morsels can bring on a horrible attack. Of course, I am just kidding. The truth is, it's bubble tea!"

Levity was a tool that he refused to part ways with. Sincerely, despite being very open about his condition, he was somewhat cautious about what information he divulged to his clients. The last thing he wanted them to do was catastrophize and impose upon themselves a diagnosis of MS because they had similar symptoms. When it comes to health, there is often a broad divide separating subjective complaints and clinical signs.

November 2006. This was Lobio's first memorable event related to MS. It occurred long before his diagnosis. Perhaps this was a clinically isolated syndrome (CIS) as described in the MS literature. A CIS was known to be an initial neurological episode.

It could be caused by inflammation or demyelination. Lobio had been feeling tired and somewhat distant for a couple weeks. On that day, he became especially symptomatic. It was lunchtime and he was jogging on the treadmill. Being able to exercise and use the equipment at work was a perk of working in a physiotherapy setting. While he was on the treadmill, he felt a sudden wave of panic, shortness of breath, and general weakness. He sat down and one of his co-workers checked his blood pressure. It was unusually high. He was also breathing rapidly. He decided it would be best to end his workday. He wanted to go home. The same co-worker graciously drove him home and almost immediately, Christine drove him to the emergency department of a local hospital. By then, his symptoms were ameliorating. While in the ER, he was examined and underwent various investigations, ultimately ruling out a cardiac episode. At the conclusion of the assessment, he was advised that he may have a flu bug and not to be surprised if he "blew chunks" later that night. This happened on a Thursday. He was advised by the ER doctor to take Friday off work. He did and started to feel better.

He never did throw up. He went back to work on Monday but unfortunately started to feel unwell again. He had thought that he was feeling well enough to return to work, but he was wrong. Despite this feeling of unease, he continued to work, and did his best. But he went home early again that day and took Tuesday off. He worked the rest of the week and went back to the ER on Saturday. Lobio explained that he had presented the previous week and he simply was not feeling better. A more detailed examination ensued, and blood was drawn to be tested. He recalled even being examined for mononucleosis. Everything came back negative. He took this as positive news despite still feeling skeptical and unwell. He was advised that he was probably battling some sort of virus and would simply have to fight it off. Only time would reveal if this were a CIS and a potential precursor to a diagnosis of MS.

Over the course of the next six months, Lobio simply did not feel himself. He felt tired, lethargic, and found himself craving sleep. While at work, he would sneak away for ten to fifteen minutes to take a catnap. When he returned home from work, he went right to bed and cozied up under the covers to sleep before dinner. He stopped playing soccer; those who knew him best knew that soccer was like a drug to him. Social gatherings simply did not appeal to him. About this time, he also noted that he was developing an intention tremor in his thumbs and index fingers, especially on the right. What was going on? Was it nothing more than something in his head? Or perhaps it really was something organic in his head. He began to do what everyone did when they are facing a health dilemma. He turned to the internet.

Diabetes. Underactive thyroid. ALS. Huntington's Chorea. Generalized anxiety disorder. These were examples of conditions that mimicked some of the symptoms he was experiencing. He convinced himself in the end that he was experiencing anxiety and that those earlier visits to the emergency department were the result of panic attacks. After approximately six months, he felt almost instantly better. No longer did he experience the same fatigue. He was working at full capacity. He resumed playing soccer. He still experienced an intention tremor in his thumbs, but this was no big deal. In fact, he consulted a neurologist in the summer of 2007, and was diagnosed with benign essential tremor, a condition that, like MS could, also resulted in involuntary shaking of a body part with movement but was not associated with any serious illness. Lobio could deal with this.

Another seven years went by with no obvious changes in his condition. Or were there? There was an episode of tinnitus in his left ear which lasted for approximately two weeks. Tinnitus is the sudden sense of often constant noise in one or both ears. For Lobio, there was a persistent humming that was simply inescapable. He was thankful that this faded but it did not completely disappear. There was also an episode of numbness and "pins and needles" in his right big toe and left inner forearm which really did not interfere with his function. There were bladder issues that could be attributed to an aging prostate, perhaps occurring a little earlier than in most men. Nonetheless, his bladder, kidney, and prostate were investigated with no obvious findings. He recalled the day when he underwent an ultrasound of these organs. He was positioned on his side, wearing a gown, but otherwise exposed to the world. The technician proceeded to ultrasound his prostate. Always fun. The technician then inquired, "Aren't you a physio?"

"What? Was it that obvious?"

Lobio was hoping that she recognized him by his face. From this examination, it was concluded that his bladder, kidneys, and prostate were clear. Once again, this was good news. He carried on with day-to-day activities while experiencing some mild inconveniences that did not really interfere with his level of function. He was getting older, with several age-related changes. Or so it seemed. In hindsight, was something inside him saying "Hello." A quote from Julius Caesar came to mind: "As a rule, men worry more about what they can't see than about what they can."

October 2013. It was a Wednesday night. Lobio remembered this because in the fall and winter he would play indoor soccer regularly with a group of his summer-league teammates and friends. He customarily played soccer all year long. While inside the gymnasium, he often played wearing an old pair of prescription glasses he did not worry about damaging. His disposable contact lenses were reserved for outdoor soccer. About midway through the two-hour session, Lobio experienced a rather sudden change in the vision of his left eye. He was perceiving a glow in that eye. He essentially lost contrast vision. Dark was bleeding into light and vice versa. He removed his glasses and examined the lens for smudging. The lens was fine. When he sat down on the bench, he covered his right eye with his hand, both with his glasses on and with them off. He was still seeing a glow. He told the others that he was experiencing strange symptoms with his vision and that he was going to go to the washroom to check his eye out in the mirror. One of his teammates said that somebody should go with him as he joked, "He might be having a stroke."

As it turned out, Lobio was not having a stroke. He resumed playing and was able to manage despite this change in vision. His right eye was fine. Despite some perceptual changes in the left, he returned home and by the time he was out of his car, his vision had normalized. He brushed the event off and soon forgot about it.

When he played floor hockey the following evening, and soccer again the following week, he experienced the same transient change in vision in his left eye. Enough was enough. He should consult his ophthalmologist. Soon afterwards, he scheduled an appointment. Based on his examination, the doctor concluded that Lobio needed a new prescription and that there were no obvious signs of eye damage or dysfunction. Lobio obtained new glasses. He used them regularly and despite seeing better at rest or during activities that were not strenuous, he still experienced the same intermittent visual deficit in his left eye. Something else was going on. What was it?

Once again Lobio turned to the internet. He knew very little about eye disease. He only knew that he was experiencing the same symptoms when he played soccer or floor hockey. He searched many conditions. Glaucoma. Macular degeneration. Cataracts. None of the symptoms related to these conditions seemed to match his profile.

Through some pensive moments, he recalled a condition called "optic neuritis" and researched it. Optic neuritis implied inflammation of the optic nerve. This nerve transmits signals from the eye to the region of the brain responsible for vision. Despite not experiencing memorable pain behind the affected eye, which was often a symptom of this condition, there were other symptoms that he did experience. Most notably, he experienced a sudden change in vision with exercise. He became aware, through his symptoms and the literature, that the change was not because of exercise; it was attributed to heat. Exercise would often increase core body temperature and thereby it often exacerbated the symptoms associated with optic neuritis. Remarkably, Lobio realized that a prolonged hot bath or shower would trigger this same response in his vision. As soon as he cooled off, the vision of his left eye would recover. He wanted to understand how and why this was happening.

Lobio found himself intrigued by optic neuritis. Through further research he came across a physiological response referred to as Uhthoff's phenomenon. It essentially identified that an increase in core body temperature, by as little as 0.5 degrees Celsius, could impair nerve conduction even further in a demyelinating condition.

"What? Demyelinating condition?"

Myelin is an insulating fatty sheath enveloping nerve cells and is essential for healthy nerve conduction. Further research of this phenomenon seemed to link these symptoms to one condition: MS.

This was not a revelation that Lobio was prepared for. A major bout of unexplained, long-lasting fatigue in 2006, with a couple visits to the ER. An episode of tinnitus of the left ear. Bladder issues consistent with urinary hesitancy and frequency. "Pins and needles" as well as numbness of the right big toe and left inner forearm. An intention tremor of the thumbs and index fingers. Now an apparent Uhthoff's phenomenon of the left eye. It was also noteworthy that his reflexes, especially in his legs, were brisk. Lobio had identified this back in his physical therapy studies when he and his classmates were practicing on each other with a reflex hammer. "Stand back or you will sustain a black eye," he would command his partner.

Either he had many separate and unrelated neurological impairments or all of them were interconnected and consistent with a larger process. The latter seemed more and more likely.

Lobio was determined to pursue this further. He did not want to delay, and he wanted definitive answers. In his mind and in his heart, he had MS, but at the same time he did not want to self-diagnose. He consulted his family physician, who listened carefully to everything Lobio had to say. He advised, "Let's order some imaging (MRI) to rule things out and we will go from there."

Lobio underwent not one but two MRIs. They were a week apart in May 2015. He obtained the results soon afterwards. There were several lesions consistent with demyelinating plaques. The conclusion of the report stated: "Suspect multiple sclerosis." Lobio seemed to be getting the answers he had been seeking for quite some time. It was bittersweet.

In July 2015, Lobio consulted his ophthalmologist once again and reported his visual symptoms. He had garnered a better understanding regarding the effect of heat on his vision. Subjectively, he reported to his ophthalmologist that it appeared as though he was experiencing Uhthoff's phenomenon. Lobio also advised him that he recently underwent two MRIs of his head and MS was suspected. When they discussed his vision, Lobio presumed that clinical tests conducted at rest would not provide any supportive findings. However, if Lobio were to play a game of soccer and then have his vision analyzed, there may be some definitive changes. His ophthalmologist concurred and had an idea. He set up a visual field test at rest and after a twenty-minute hard run. Lobio ran around the neighbourhood where the clinic was situated. He heated up and then immediately completed a visual field test. The results confirmed that he was indeed experiencing Uhthoff's phenomenon. After the run, Lobio could not see the test's dots as well with his left eye. Later that month Lobio consulted a neuro-ophthalmologist, who reviewed his MRI reports. He also completed some tests of his own. He pulled up one of Lobio's MRIs, and by changing the contrast of the image, he was able to identify scarring on Lobio's left optic nerve. This could point to a demyelinating process. He concluded that Lobio could be dealing with signs and symptoms consistent with MS, but he could not make any guarantees. He referred Lobio to the MS clinic.

As Lobio waited five months for his appointment in January 2016, he noticed new symptoms. He was becoming more unsteady on his feet. He did not notice this when he walked leisurely or with purpose. However, when he played soccer, he was experiencing Uhthoff's phenomenon with respect to his dynamic balance, instead of his left eye as in the year before. In other words, the longer that he played soccer, the more unsteady he became. He was experiencing a feeling of drunkenness. He felt like he was trying to walk on a rocking boat. He knew that if he were to encounter a sobriety check and complete the walking component after leaving soccer, he would undoubtedly fail. Remarkably, his visual symptoms had resolved about one year after they started. With his balance, within ten to fifteen minutes after playing soccer and cooling off, he became steady again.

Around this time, Lobio also began to experience what felt like an electric shock in his lower spine and pelvic region when he nodded his head to look at the floor. This was consistent with Lhermitte's sign and another clinical sign of MS. Keeping in mind his clinical signs, subjective complaints, and MRI reports, this was certainly looking a lot like one sinister culprit. Lobio was fortunate to be getting the answers he was looking for, but he was also distressed that everything was pointing to one common denominator: multiple sclerosis.

A Bad Dream
Becomes a Reality

January 2016. Lobio was forty-three years old and would soon be turning forty-four. "It would appear that you have MS." This was the first time that a doctor said this to Lobio. Based on his symptoms, clinical signs, and MRI findings, he had felt for some time that this dreaded diagnosis was inevitable. However, everything became a reality on that day. He became "Lobio, the guy with MS." Everything that he had and everything that he had worked for became secondary, at least to him.

His appointment on that day was scheduled for two o'clock. His neurologist worked out of a hospital two hours away from his hometown. Since the appointment was later in the day, Lobio decided to work in the morning. For quite some time, he had been working as a physiotherapist in a private clinic as well as at the hospital. On that morning, he was scheduled to work at the clinic. It was a relatively uneventful morning. He decided to work so that he could distance his thoughts from his pending medical appointment. Christine picked him up at eleven and they immediately headed down the highway.

The drive was a long and somewhat monotonous one. The topography was flat and, given the time of year, the leaves had abandoned the trees. Farmland, farmhouses, cars, transport trucks, overpasses, and intermittent windmills passed by. Lobio was entirely distracted. As a passenger, he found himself staring aimlessly through the window and upward toward the sparsely clouded sky. An occasional hawk circled overhead. Lobio's thoughts were elsewhere. Without warning, he teared up and started to cry. He could not be consoled. He was preparing for the inevitable. He was preparing for those words from the doctor who he was yet to meet. Christine grasped his hand. She didn't say anything because she didn't know what to say.

"Christine, I love you. I'm scared. Let's turn around and go back home. I just need to soak in the tub. It will all be better then."

These words were not enough to persuade her to turn around. Lobio and Christine arrived at the campus of the university hospital. They proceeded to the Neurosciences Department. He was introduced to his neurologist and a nurse practitioner. He had prepared by bringing a complete list of his symptoms. They had access to Lobio's MRI reports dating back to May 2015. They also had the reports from his family physician and his neuro-ophthalmologist. He was gifted with a thorough assessment. "It would appear that you have MS." What Lobio was not prepared for was: "It tends to be more aggressive in males and you should go on medication." Once again, the reality hit him hard. Lobio had thought he was going to be advised to carry on with normal life and that he would be monitored. This was not the case. He had some big decisions to make.

Lobio was ultimately diagnosed with MS of the relapsing-remitting type. On the advice of his neurologist, he decided to start disease-modifying therapy. He would begin treatment in the spring. The medication was not designed to alleviate his symptoms but rather to mitigate future flare-ups. Lobio accepted his current level of function and he could live with this.

Lobio's mother was one of the first people that he shared this information with. She wore a look of disbelief and despair. She stated, "Maybe this is my fault." She teared up.

"Why you?" people would often ask. "Why not?" was Lobio's response.

This was life.

Underestimating Multiple Sclerosis

In time, Lobio realized that he had miscalculated MS's ferocity. What he learned in school and at work paled in comparison to what he felt. He carried on with normal life for a while but eventually the disease began to chip away at him. The disease was especially aggressive in the first few years. Initially it was soccer. The more he ran, the more he heated up. With heat came unsteadiness and clumsiness. With that came more time on the sidelines. Eventually that became frustrating. Soccer was so close yet so far. His teammates were always supportive, but opposing players were unaware of his plight.

"Nice dive," he would hear, knowing it was the disease that made him fall.

Despite not playing as much or at all, he was still a part of the team, at least to his teammates. Lobio was encouraged by his teammates to join them for the post-game handshake with the opposing team. "Good game, even though you didn't do anything," said one opposing player.

"I've been told that I was a pretty good soccer player not that long ago." Lobio just shook his head.

That player's comment discouraged Lobio from joining the team for handshakes thereafter.

Leaving the comfort of his home to attend concerts or sporting events also became inconvenient and stressful. Eventually the reward was not worth the risk. He was able to walk, but not well and not for long distances. The need to go to the washroom frequently was also another consideration that instilled anxiousness. If he did attend an event, he refrained from drinking . . . anything. Once, at a Red Wings–Maple Leafs game, Lobio had stumbled over someone's foot while attempting to shuffle to his seat midway down the row.

"Have another," the fan remarked as he stood cradling his beer.

"I'm sorry about that," Lobio replied. He thought to himself: "I have not even had one. Now I need one."

Travelling also posed similar questions. How far is it? Is it a drive or a flight? How much walking is required? Who is going? Will someone be there to help? How close are the washrooms? The questions went on and on. Christine and Lobio were planning a trip to Italy. Christine was speaking with a representative from a tour company over the phone.

"Your husband will hold us all up. This is not a good tour for him."

"It's true. Please help us out. Give us options. There must be some. Or maybe there isn't."

When Christine told Lobio about this conversation, he felt defeated. He did not know how to respond.

"I guess it's my (our) problem," he thought.

On the rare occasion that Lobio went out in public, there was often no shortage of frustration. He and Christine were enjoying their anniversary dinner at a local restaurant when a group of eight sat next to them. The individual who joined the group last came in, removed his coat, placed it on the back of the chair, and took a seat. He was clearly rushed. When he sat down, he was laughing and boasted to the others, "There weren't any close parking spots left so I parked in a handicapped spot. I guess I'm an asshole." He continued to laugh.

"Yes, you are," Lobio thought to himself.

Lobio's life was falling to pieces. Playing soccer in the backyard with Andrew . . . gone. Going for a run . . . gone. Going for a long walk . . . gone. Attending social events . . . gone. Drinking more than one beer at a time . . . gone. Getting dressed or completing activities of daily living standing up . . . gone. A steady right hand . . . gone. Legible writing . . . gone. A peaceful, uninterrupted night of sleep . . . gone. Smiling . . . gone.

Then there was work.

The Inevitable Collision
of Two Worlds

For many dealing with a chronic health condition, work can offer a much-needed escape. As a physiotherapist surrounded by individuals with MS and other debilitating neurological conditions, it was not an escape for Lobio. By contrast, it was a heavy reminder. His body alerted him to what MS was doing. His eyes revealed to him what MS could do. In fact, often what he saw exacerbated what he felt. He wanted to remain at work, but he would often weigh the pros and cons. He had honestly believed that he would be able to remain employed in the same capacity that he was accustomed to. In his mind, he would complete his career working two busy jobs: one in the public sector and one in the private sector. Both were very rewarding physically, mentally, and financially.

Initially he sacrificed hours at the clinic. While maintaining full-time employment at the hospital, Lobio was still able to manage part-time hours at the private clinic. The work at the hospital was more manageable as the pace was slower. As time went on, he realized that he needed to step away even more. Reluctantly, he eventually gave up part-time work at the clinic. His plan was to take a break for a few months and then return. He relinquished the income that he was accustomed to, but he realized that this did not blemish the bigger picture. Both he and his family would not only manage fine, but they would be better for it.

In conjunction with giving up work at the clinic altogether, Lobio also cut his hours down at the hospital. His hours were reduced by half, for three months. It appeared that the disease was winning. However, he hoped that this time off would serve him well and provide him with an opportunity to refresh his body and mind. He could give more of himself in all aspects of life by reducing his hours at work. His family and co-workers supported his decision, perhaps more than he supported himself.

After some much-needed rest, Lobio resumed his full-time hours at the hospital. He was refreshed and was realizing the benefits of a strong course of steroids. Despite having many ongoing symptoms, he experienced overall improvement, both subjectively and objectively. He was eating better. He maintained a relatively active lifestyle while respecting his limitations. He was regaining control. Everyone around him stated that he looked better and he seemed to be managing better.

Lobio managed to effectively do his job but unfortunately the following year he fell victim to another exacerbation—the worst yet. His neurologist recommended that he change from his current disease-modifying medication to a more aggressive one. Lobio initiated this treatment at the end of the summer. This medication was designed to suppress his immune system, with the goal of curbing self-attack on his central nervous system. Unfortunately, he became more vulnerable to other pathogens. Upper respiratory tract infections were not uncommon with this medication, and Lobio was no exception. Often, he felt he was battling a cold. If he was not on God's radar before this medication, he certainly was afterwards, as there was never a shortage of "God bless you" in his daily life. In mid-October he noticed a few water blisters on the left side of his trunk. Shingles. Yet another obstacle. His neurological symptoms amplified. Walking became even more difficult. He began using a cane. Then he switched to a forearm crutch. Was this setback transient or was it an actual change in his condition for the worse?

Lobio cut down his work hours even more through the support of his family physician. Initially he tried working reduced hours as he had done the previous fall and winter. After three weeks of doing this, he reached the point where he was just dragging his body. It was difficult for him to focus. Lobio was in a noticeably weaker state, and distant. He was not reliable. One day he would work, one day he would call in sick. This was neither fair to his clients nor to his co-workers.

It was a brisk day in November and the leaves were falling from the trees. Lobio, too, felt that he was falling. Perhaps he would just fall and wither away. He trudged into work with his right foot catching on the ground with every step. He relied so heavily on his crutch that he was surprised it didn't bow and snap in half. He had reached his limit as he was succumbing to this terrible disease. He laboured through his shift and realized that he was of no good to the clients who he was serving, nor to himself. He deduced that he was ineffective as a physiotherapist. Lobio recognized that he was fragile and that he was broken. He needed to take some time off work once again. As much as he wanted to fight this notion and remain defiant to this disease, it had other thoughts. He followed his heart. He was pushing himself to the limit. Later that day, at half past four, Lobio punched out for the last time, at least for a while.

In addition to the support that Lobio received from his family physician, he was also backed by the hospital occupational health nurse. He was tentatively scheduled to remain off work for approximately twelve weeks. It was the best possible decision for all parties involved. His co-workers graciously took on his caseload. "Go home. Stay home for a while. We've got this."

"Goodbye for now. I hope that I return a more reliable co-worker and physiotherapist."

Lobio realized that he was giving up a daily driving force. He was also giving up, at least temporarily, the physical and emotional support that his occupation offered. Now, he would be even more on his own and he would need to remain diligent, purposeful, and smart if he was going to ensure that this time off would be beneficial. He needed to address physical, mental, emotional, and spiritual needs and, most importantly, the relationships in his life.

A Dark Path

There was no BEEP! BEEP! BEEP! BEEP! BEEP! There was no need to wake up for anything in a timely manner except to ensure that the kids got themselves up and ready for school. In fact, Lobio could direct them as he lay in bed. During the initial two weeks of his time off, he fell deeper into oblivion. It became commonplace for him to wake up late, lollygag, eat whenever, and drown in meaningless television, all the while waiting for his family to arrive home. Lobio hit rock bottom. He was closing the shades. One day, he was relaxing on the couch downstairs watching TV with Christine sitting next to him. She was folding laundry.

"How are you?" she asked.

"My symptoms are not too bad today. I think I slept well," Lobio answered.

"That's good. But really, how are you doing?"

Lobio knew what she was getting at. Tears immediately began to well up in his eyes.

He said, "Sometimes I wish I could just fall asleep and never wake up again."

The thought of ending his life had never entered Lobio's mind. It was instead a feeling of indifference. "Whatever. Who cares? It doesn't matter what I say or do. Or what anyone says or does for that matter. I thought I had this thing under control. I was wrong. I feel like an iron "M" is shackled to my right ankle and an "S" to my left. I am treading water in the middle of the ocean. I should just let myself slip under. Drowning seems inevitable. It will all be over soon. MS, you win. I lose. I hope you're happy. Actually, I don't."

His attitude and motivation were changing for the worse. He had never conveyed this apathy to his clients as he had always provided physiotherapy to the best of his abilities. This thinking was more reflective of all other aspects of his life. When he woke up in the morning, his first thought was that he had MS. He could feel MS. He would get out of bed and take his first few steps. His body reminded him of this reality. As the day went on, everything that he did, either at work or at home, he managed in his own way knowing and feeling he had MS. When he went to bed in the evening, he tried to fall asleep ignoring the fact that he had MS, but it was very difficult. It was so distracting. When he remembered his dreams, he was playing soccer. He was running and jumping. He was walking unimpeded and without thought. Then he would wake up. These dreams had become his nightmares. He was not dreaming about pain, suffering, fear, or desperation. They were dreams about functional activities that he used to excel at and often took for granted. When he eventually woke up, he was back to his MS reality. It was a repetitive, monotonous cycle of misery.

"Maybe I won't go to sleep tonight. These disheartening dreams are tormenting me. I know that I need sleep, but my mind seems to be waiting for me to drift off so it can give me false hope. And then I wake up and fall flat on my face."

Lobio felt he had given all of himself in life and he had nothing more to give. In the past, he had overcome many challenging obstacles that were beyond his control. He came out on top and became a much better person as a result. Now he had been dealt this massive blow and it was nothing short of overwhelming. It often held him prisoner.

After witnessing the grievous impact that mental health challenges could have on a person, Lobio once disclosed to a co-worker, "I would rather lose my legs than lose my mind." Now here he was, losing his legs, and it was making him lose his mind. Dealing with loss after loss wore Lobio down. He realized that it was not a physical death that he feared. What he did fear was the death of the future he had envisioned and, sooner or later, the death of his dreams. His goals and aspirations needed to change. He wanted to change how he saw the world. Lobio became committed to embrace his new reality.

A Peaceful Surrender

Lobio eventually learned to respect MS. However, he had given it too much credit. "I am MS and I have Lobio," he thought. With his wife's help, Lobio came to another realization. Christine commented, "I feel you are only happy when you are miserable." Lobio concurred. She was right. There was a time when he was happy. There was a time when he looked at the positive and felt optimistic. What happened to that guy? He recovered well from other life crises. Why not this one? He was still trying to figure this out. He wanted to be the Lobio of old.

Curbing negative thoughts and emotions as well as avoiding temptations came first. Where he had failed most and what he had been preoccupied with was the notion of how others perceived him. For far too long, Lobio placed the views of others well above the views he had of himself. This realization did not strike him in the gut with a sudden fury. It was the culmination of many observations and pensive moments. Self-reflection was the cornerstone of his survival. For one, he recognized that he needed to part ways with his own bravado.

"I will have pain. I will have weakness. I will be unsteady. I will be clumsy. The weather will affect me. I will cry at times. I will need to be alone sometimes. I am mortal. I will deal with my new reality. Before I die, I want to live."

It was essential that he also stop feeling entitled. He would benefit most from humbling himself to this disease as it would be the only way to live with it. This did not mean giving up. It meant transforming his own frustration and pride into cooperation with MS and driving to push himself both physically and mentally.

Lobio had been seeking acceptance ever since his diagnosis. In fact, looking back, perhaps he accepted this diagnosis too soon and he underestimated its potential to alter his life plan. When he was asking others to be patient with him and understand why he did things the way that he did, he was speaking to himself. He had to accept a life with limitations, different responsibilities, and new expectations. Through his work as a physiotherapist, he had witnessed all too often that those who accepted their own diagnoses and limitations were better able to move forward and physically rehabilitate themselves. Those who denied that they would have limitations struggled more to achieve realistic goals.

"I want to golf like I did when I was thirty," said the eighty-year-old retired businessman. He complained of right shoulder pain and he was referred to Lobio for physiotherapy.

"If that is his goal, then I have already failed before I have even laid a hand on him."

MS was not a terminal diagnosis, but it certainly was a game-changer. In some ways, Lobio supposed that it could be likened to a loss of life while not quite reaching death. Death sat at the peak of the mountain. Sadly, there were times that he had hoped that the mountain would become inverted so that he could accelerate toward the peak.

Like any chronic illness, MS commanded surrender, followed by discipline. Yet it was so unpredictable, with no two individuals sharing this diagnosis following the same course. It could make its presence known with a quiet whisper and culminate with nothing more than a numb finger for over seventy years of life. By contrast, it could make its presence known with a thunderous roar as an individual could become wheelchair-bound in the blink of an eye. No matter the type of MS, the person with this unfortunate diagnosis remained in a constant state of wonderment. Waiting for something yet hoping for nothing. MS would sit back and tuck itself away, like a deadly viper camouflaged behind a bush, preparing to ambush an unwary mouse.

Lobio was arrogant and ignorant when he was diagnosed. This disease had gradually chipped away at him physically, mentally, and emotionally. Now, he was driven to plan more for the future because he didn't know what was in store. He didn't want to be afraid. He needed to stop catastrophizing.

"This disease is not a joke. Nothing will come easy anymore, but I will be ok."

Negative emotions, he learned, would rile this disease. He had paid dearly. Jealousy—he had been there. There were many times that he found himself overanalyzing those around him. He would compare his situation to theirs. He would see things that people had that he ultimately wanted. He would see them walking down the sidewalk and he wanted that. He saw them looking up and around without losing their balance and he wanted that. He saw them playing sports or talking about the sports that they played over the weekend and he wanted that.

"Look at that guy crossing the street. His clothes don't fit well, and he looks so disheveled. He is taking steps ever so effortlessly and is probably thinking about what's for dinner. *No.* Stop it. Don't be that way. He exudes self-confidence in his own way. Where he is coming from and where he is going, I don't know. He is walking with purpose. He is being active. His ability to walk is a gift and he has chosen to use that gift. I am happy for him now."

"Look at that out of shape forty-year-old father of three on the soccer field. A couple of his kids play the game, so he has decided to give soccer a try having never played before. He can hardly run ten meters without becoming short of breath. When the ball is coming at his upper body he panics as if it were a grenade. He uses his hands to defend himself. That's a no-no. His five-year-old son probably kicks better than him with his non-dominant foot. *No*. Stop it. Don't be that way. He is having a great time. He is smiling and laughing. He is being active. He is understanding the game now and he is improving. He is a great team player. I respect him. I am very happy for him."

Lobio also became absorbed with self-pity. This had adverse consequences in all aspects of his life. This emotion led Lobio down the path of isolation. Even when he was physically present, he was not there. Feeling sorry for himself, and complaining, drove people even further away. Maybe this was what he was trying to do, yet, he wanted them back. He needed them.

Lobio also realized that he had a short fuse. Everything seemed to make him angry. Anger is not uncommon in those suffering from MS. There are many triggers. The loss of function and the fear of future regression could be triggers. He needed to let things go. Lobio especially came to this realization in a moment he shared with his mother. He invited her to accompany him to one of his neurologist appointments. During this time together, they became engaged in some deeper conversation. His mother told Lobio what he needed to hear. She told him that he had every right to be distressed about his current situation. However, she felt that he was letting little things get to him too much. She wanted him to focus on what was important and let the rest go. She advised him that this would be one of the best ways to deal with MS. This drive home was a valuable turning point for Lobio. It was not a long drive home after all. In fact, it was too short.

The fact that Lobio had MS and needed help more than antici-pated only amplified life's minor irritations and how they impacted him. Lobio didn't want to ask for help but he needed to. He became enlightened by the countless people in his life who were helping him through this. He needed to focus on this and appreciate this. He realized that his way was not necessarily the best way. He needed to let the little things go. For example, situations that he perceived to be untidy, such as shoes not being neatly put away at the front entrance, or a drawer left open. Not only would he be better for it, but those around him would become more comfortable in his company. He wanted to enjoy life and he wanted those who loved him to feel comfortable around him.

Lobio ultimately realized that honesty served him much better than hiding his emotions. "I am not ok. But I am doing my best." That was the answer to Lobio's least favourite question: "How are you?" He could lie and say that he was okay but what benefit would there be to that? Maybe it was what people wanted to hear but he felt they could see right through him, especially those who knew him best. Being open and blunt served him well. It shaped the beginning of a positive transformation.

Discovering a More Compatible Reality

Lobio was lying in bed and gazing up at the ceiling fan as it rotated endlessly. He became pensive. The time had come to live anew. The wheels were spinning. Once again, he was planning a different future. He didn't just need to get better. He wanted to get better.

Firstly, Lobio needed to identify what "getting better" meant. Did it mean that he would suddenly get up and walk effortlessly? Did it mean that he would run? Did it mean that he would not have to think about how often he would be required to go up and down the stairs? Most importantly, did it mean that he would be seen in public without his crutch? If the answer to any of these questions was "yes," then he had already failed.

Secondly, Lobio needed to establish goals that were both realistic and attainable. As this disease was unpredictable and could strike anywhere within the central nervous system, he would take it upon himself to stimulate his body and mind in ways that not only battled the progression but also, he hoped, would promote positive change. It was well-established that the brain was very plastic and through creative and repetitive stimulation, new electrical pathways could be formed within the healthy nervous system tissue (Doidge, 2007). He identified several activities and factors that warranted his attention.

Sleep was one such activity. Lobio craved a solid night of sleep. He appreciated this fundamental need and learned not to underestimate its value. Sleep was *Il paradiso dei poveri*: the paradise of the poor, as his father used to say.

Lobio looked forward to sleep yet also feared its approach. Like arising in the morning, it was often at that moment just before falling asleep that he was most reminded of this disease. The ineluctable symptoms were at the forefront of his mind just prior to falling asleep. Spasticity, neuropathy, twitching, and unwanted speculation were ingredients for an unsavoury plate of insomnia. It was at this time he found medication to be of greatest benefit. A circulating fan, especially blowing air over his feet, offered some comfort. A solid night of sleep was vital to his performance the following day.

Lobio learned to dread an increase in his body temperature. Most people looked forward to the comfort offered by a warm bath, a crackling fire in the fireplace, or a restful nap outside on a hot summer day. Lobio loved these activities but it was not mutual. Heat did not love him back. In fact, it only reminded him more of MS.

The DC Comics superhero *Superman,* created by Jerry Siegel and Joe Shuster, first appeared on the cover of Action Comics #1 in June 1938. He was immobilized and brought down to his knees by the artificial substance called *krytonite.*

Heat had become Lobio's kryptonite. Specifically, an increase in body temperature could prompt a transient worsening of some, if not all his symptoms. Humidity would further exacerbate his situation. Fatigue worsened. He even had to visit the washroom more often. He felt increased numbness over patchy areas of his body and his skin would burn. He became so ataxic and unsteady on his feet that from the point of view of an outsider, it looked like he had partied a little too hard. This was a classic case of Uhthoff's phenomenon. This seemed like an easy problem to solve. "Stay cool and I will be fine," he thought. In fact, it was not so simple. He could sit inside behind a fan all day but was that how it would be for the remainder of his life? He wanted to take a warm bath. He wanted to ride his bike. He wanted to go outside on a hot summer day to barbecue some steaks. Was he willing to pay the price of engaging in these activities? The answer was yes; the enjoyment of these simple pleasures was worth some discomfort later. Usually.

Lobio recalled one ill-fated evening when he just could not seem to warm up. He had taken his disease-modifying medication, which was known to give him the chills and a slight fever. In addition to this, he was also feeling a little under the weather. He indulged in an extra-long hot bath. Afterwards, he draped himself in his housecoat and went to bed under a few layers of blankets. He awoke in the middle of the night, overheated and sweaty. He was burning up. He was overwhelmed with a deep sense of urgency. He had to get to the bathroom, and soon.

Lobio reluctantly hurried out of bed and proceeded to the bathroom with an extra-large base of support between his feet. He was leaning heavily on the walls. He entered the bathroom, switched on the lights, turned his body, and immediately stumbled forward, unable to steady himself. He came crashing down onto the toilet. It cracked open like an egg. Water was suddenly spraying everywhere like a geyser. He had never seen Old Faithful in Yellowstone National Park, but he had a miniature version of it in his bathroom. Christine heard the commotion. She jumped out of bed and came to his aid. Lobio was able to rise from his position on the broken toilet but he was drenched with toilet water. He was very upset, but not because of the mess—he still had to relieve himself and the other bathroom was in the basement. "Stairs. Crap."

Anyhow, Lobio made it. He had also learned a valuable lesson. Prior to returning to bed, he changed his clothes. He remained uncovered, with the fan blowing over him at full speed. Upon awakening in the morning, he was back to his normal baseline.

Lobio had come to the realization that cooling would essentially offset the heat and normalize his core temperature such that nerve conduction would be at its peak. In other words, the myriad of symptoms that were exacerbated by heat were reduced when he cooled off.

Data suggests that a vast majority of those with MS experience a worsening of symptoms which is also evident clinically with an increase in core body temperature. Lobio researched why this would happen. He came across a couple of theories. One was that heat could impair nerve conduction at the level of the neuron. Another was that lesions of the hypothalamus, a tiny structure in the midbrain, could impair thermoregulation, the body's ability to maintain a relatively stable core temperature within different environments and conditions. Whatever the reason, heat was a potent adversary, at least for Lobio.

What could he do to eliminate the heat and the humidity outside? Absolutely nothing. Mother Nature made her own rules. She was the self-appointed CEO of the natural world and efforts to change her mind would always be futile. If it was a warm day and he needed to be outside for an extended period, he would seek shade. He would also wear clothing that breathed. If he was sitting on the backyard deck, he could have a fan blowing on him if there was no breeze. Finally, he could return indoors where the air was cooler.

Indoors, there were many solutions. Air conditioning. Fans. A cool shower or bath. "I'm home so my shirt is coming off. I suppose I better keep it on at work."

Could he take a hot shower or bath? Absolutely. However, he knew that this would pose a risk. His functional abilities would be impaired afterwards. He would often "wash" the heat off himself with cool water at the conclusion of a hot bath or shower. This would work wonders.

What about exercise? He had to move. Everyone needed to move. He had always been active. Why stop now? In fact, now was the time to move even more than he used to as it was the first line of defense against this incessant bully. He needed to be smart as to where, when, and how he exercised. He could ride the living daylights out of his bike inside while it was mounted on a trainer. He would undoubtedly be in disarray afterwards, but he knew that it would be short-lived. A great deal of planning went into riding his bike outdoors, but it could be done. It often depended on the temperature and weather, but so be it. He could pace himself and rest as needed so his body heat did not have the opportunity to accumulate. There were also cooling vests which he understood could be very effective. He was planning on investigating them further.

Lobio became committed to discovering new pastimes. Without a functional pair of legs, he felt especially lost. Soccer had become a fleeting memory, and this had been difficult for Lobio to accept. He had been certain that he would be able to play for many more years. Perhaps no other activity in his life reminded him more of his loss than soccer. He missed the weekly ritual and he missed his teammates.

Despite no longer being able to play, Lobio still loved the game and it remained a meaningful part of his life. "If I am not going to play on my team, then I am going to watch them play."

Lobio often rode his bike to their venue. Sometimes the rides were up to thirty-five kilometers one way. He had benefited from some exercise in his own way. He would even help the team from the sidelines. His teammates wanted him around and he eventually found ways to contribute.

Playing vicariously in Andrew's soccer boots also gave him great satisfaction. Andrew had grown to love the sport. He played to enjoy the game. Lobio would coach him in the backyard or on the pitch. He watched his son's skills evolve. Andrew's footwork was better than Lobio's ever was. It was important that Andrew knew that Lobio was there by his side when he played and that his dad was encouraging his every move. Lobio was proud of him.

Lobio also engaged in new hobbies. Reading and subsequently writing were stimulating and therapeutic. He had never taken the time to appreciate their value before. He found that reading classic works provided him with an insightful perspective of the past and present. They even bolstered him as he dealt with MS. His own writing evolved. He became a big fan of words. Lobio knew that there would always be ways to play!

As an adjunct to riding his bike, Lobio needed to discover other ways to exercise. The possibilities were endless.

"Hurt versus harm." Back in physical therapy school, this philosophy became a cornerstone of theory. In other words, exercise sometimes produced discomfort. However, this risk was outweighed by the long-term benefit. For Lobio, kneeling was an example. When he knelt, he experienced a noxious discomfort in his knees due to neuropathy. He knew he was not inflicting tissue damage, yet the sensation that he was experiencing told him otherwise. A jumbled motherboard in his head was relaying false information through a muddled circuit system down his spine and ultimately to the skin over and around his knees. It was fake but real. It was a lie but the truth. In the end, he reassured himself that he was not harming himself. He was thereby able to kneel longer. "Mind over matter."

Lobio then established what his symptoms, clinical signs, and goals were. As a physiotherapist, this is what he was required to do with each of his clients, so this is what he should do for himself.

Firstly, he wanted to traverse from point A to point B with greater ease so that he would be able to take care of whatever was needed at point B. At the time, Lobio walked to accomplish this. What exercises could facilitate this?

Spasticity was one hurdle that he was forced to confront. In the simplest terms, spasticity is an increase in muscle tone resulting in tightness of muscles and stiffness of joints. There are characteristic muscle groups of the lower extremities that are affected: the quadriceps (the large muscle group at the front of the thigh) and the gastrocnemius (the calf muscle). These muscle groups would often tighten up to evoke extension (straightening) of the lower extremities to assist a person to stand upright. Unfortunately, spasticity could become so severe that it could restrict the fluid movement of joints (for example the knee or ankle) and in some cases, it could cause a person to catch their foot when walking, creating a tripping hazard. There were ways to manage this medically, including medication and bracing, but there were also exercises that could be helpful. Regular stretching of tight muscle groups could be incorporated into a daily routine. A few repetitions held for thirty generous seconds for each major muscle group worked well to maintain flexibility and reduce spasticity. Lobio would often apply ice or moist heat to spastic muscles. Soaking in a warm bath with jacuzzi jets to circulate the water would relax tight muscles. Avoiding sitting and lying down for prolonged periods (except to sleep) also worked wonders. Lobio didn't necessarily need to get up and walk. When he would watch TV, he would stand up and shift weight toward the right and toward the left. He would set a timer and remain standing for fifteen to twenty minutes. He would also get up and down and do squats several times. This kept his muscles in check and would limit the onset of spasticity and tightness.

Lobio also needed to regain greater control of his lower extremities. His leg movements, specifically his walking pattern, had become choppy and his foot placement had become sloppy. He was trying his best to get from point A to point B and oftentimes it was not aesthetically pleasing. Lobio guessed that he would never be a runway model. Nonetheless, there were ways that he could sharpen the control of his legs. While lying on his back he would slide the heel of one foot up and down the shin of the opposite leg with his eyes open, progressing to doing this with his eyes closed. This was a fantastic control exercise that could be made more challenging by progressing to doing it in a standing position while holding onto a countertop. If standing balance was sufficient, completing this exercise unsupported would be the next logical progression. Stepping up and over pool noodles forwards, backwards, and sideways was also very effective. This exercise could be progressed by holding onto a stable piece of furniture or countertop with two hands, then one hand, then letting go altogether. Lobio also found single leg walking on a treadmill to be highly effective. With his left leg firmly planted on the side of the treadmill, he would work on step control and length with his right leg as the belt was running. He would place as little or as much weight through his right leg as he felt that he needed to. Upon completion of this exercise he would walk with both legs on the treadmill.

Lobio needed to hone his balance while both sitting and standing. People who had poor balance were at risk of falling, which could have disastrous consequences. Lobio knew there were three body systems that individuals engaged to maintain functional balance. The visual system is responsible for what people see with their eyes. The vestibular system manages what is perceived within the inner ear with respect to spatial orientation (the ability to maintain posture in relation to the surrounding environment). The somatosensory system is responsible for what is felt (pain, pressure, vibration, temperature) anywhere within the body. All three systems relay valuable information to the brain's cerebral cortex for processing. Lobio should provoke all three of these systems. He could challenge his balance by standing within the parallel bars at work with different bases of support. For example, feet close together, one foot ahead of the other, tandem standing (standing with one foot directly in front of the other), or single leg standing. He could make each of these exercises that much more difficult by closing his eyes. He would use a timer to monitor his progress. At home, he didn't have parallel bars. Consequently, he could complete these exercises with his back to a corner. With the wall on either side and a sturdy chair in front, there would be nowhere to go. It would be safe. Of course, when in doubt, he would have someone nearby.

These exercises would challenge his static balance but there would also be a dynamic component that needed to be addressed. The best way to challenge his dynamic balance was to walk. Lobio endeavoured to walk more and improve the quality of his gait. He could add or remove an assistive walking device. He could turn his head left or right or nod his head up and down as he walked. This was surprisingly difficult for him. He could walk with a trustworthy companion. One of his primary goals was to indefinitely maintain some semblance of walking.

Lobio knew he needed to maintain his strength. Traditional exercises, such as lifting weights, were of great benefit. He needed to be able to manipulate his own body so that he could essentially get from place to place or complete functional tasks and activities of daily living. Much could be accomplished without weights as he could work against his own body weight. There were sit-ups, pushups, bridges, planks, squats, lunges, transitioning from sitting to standing and vice versa, and stepping up and down on a step. There were so many creative ways to work on strength and the body would respond in a favourable way. Having said that, improvements in strength did not directly translate to improvements in walking.

Walking is a multi-coordinated task that incorporates strength, balance, and control.

How about introducing an exercise ball? Sitting, bridging, or kneeling on the ball were excellent ways to put balance, control, and strength to the test.

In relation to walking, there were certain muscle groups that needed to be maintained. The large muscle groups that kept him upright were obvious. There were the quadriceps at the front of the thigh. But how about its antagonist at the back of the thigh, the hamstrings? This muscle group would serve as the primary knee flexor. In other words, the function of this muscle was to bend the knee. But what happened when this muscle was weak and did not adequately bend the knee during the gait cycle? As a result of an unfortunate flare-up, Lobio found out. He was dragging his right leg. His right knee did not adequately flex during the swing phase of gait and he was catching his foot, thereby making him more likely to trip, wear out the tip of his shoe, or both. He targeted much attention to this muscle group, and, in time, he was rewarded with a more efficient gait pattern, no longer catching his right foot.

Moving down to the ankle and foot, these anatomical structures were the first to meet the ground during gait. As such, maintaining adequate mobility, strength, and control were of vital importance here. There were strong muscle groups at the back of the leg making up the calf. These springy muscles contributed to push-off and propelled the individual forward. They were also the primary muscles engaged when hopping or jumping. Detrimentally, they often became hypertonic (having abnormally increased muscle tone), and spastic with upper motor neuron lesions or disease. How about their antagonistic (counteracting) muscles at the front of the foot, ankle, and lower leg? In medical terms they were collectively referred to as ankle dorsiflexors. Weakness in these muscles during gait resulted in a drop foot (difficulty lifting the front aspect of the foot). This presented as another common problem in the neurologically impaired population. Combine this problem with weak hamstrings (in other words, impaired knee flexion with impaired ankle dorsiflexion), and the leg and foot would drag even more. Catching the tip of the foot on the ground often resulted. The person's gait would become highly inefficient and, in many cases, unsafe. Lobio focused on this muscle group and, in time, he was not dragging his leg to the same extent, if at all. Bracing can also help individuals who were struggling with these muscle groups. For example, an ankle-foot orthosis is a type of brace that can be used during gait to control ankle motion and counter drop foot.

There were also exercises that targeted the pelvic floor: Kegel exercises. Engaging these muscles can improve bowel and bladder control. The beauty of these exercises is that they can be completed anywhere, anytime. Just sitting around at work or watching TV, an individual can engage these muscles simply by consciously tightening the pelvic floor. It is a well-known fact that activating these muscles also engages the deep lumbar stabilizers, thus improving strength and stability of the low back. What a bonus!

For Lobio, all these exercises served an indispensable purpose. They were designed to fine-tune his body as he carried on with essential daily activities. Without this focus, his movement and control could be sloppy, and his independence could shift to dependence. His heart needed exercise too—not just emotional, but physical. It, along with the lungs, serve to pump fundamental nutrients and oxygen throughout the body via the circulatory system. He would not be doing these essential organs any justice if he did not exercise them as well. He needed to get his heart pumping and to expand his lungs. Soccer used to do this for him. Now what? Nothing got him working harder than his bike. Outside could be a challenge due to balance and coordination deficits. However, having his bike mounted on a trainer, inside, offered a safe solution. He could ride and push himself to the limit and so he did. Not only did his stamina improve, but his thighs had never been so muscular.

After a five-minute cool down following a long bike ride, he even walked better than he did before he got on the bike. A forty-five to sixty-minute ride, three times per week was something he looked forward to.

Lobio knew that everyone needed to move. That was the bottom line. The choice of when, how, and where was based on personal choice. The pros and cons should always be weighed. Whatever the sport or activity, everyone's body craved movement; not only the bones, muscles, heart, and lungs, but the brain too.

Like soccer, travelling also seemed to be but a fleeting memory. Lobio had been so privileged and seen so much of the world. He did not want the opportunities to cease because his body was not as cooperative as he desired.

"Am I trapped? Will I remain within the confines of my home or workplace from now on? Will I travel only within the borders of my city and occasionally outside of it . . . for medical appointments?"

It was Thanksgiving, 2017. It was nearly two years since he had been diagnosed. Lobio elected to ride his bike over to his sister-in-law's house. Christine's two younger sisters were both married, with children of their own. It was tradition to have Thanksgiving dinner at one of their homes. Lobio had just arrived on his bike and was sitting and cooling off in the backyard by himself. Everyone was already inside. After a few minutes, his brother-in-law came out back and he greeted him with an ice-cold beer. "How's it going?"

With that question, Lobio was speechless. He had a meltdown and started to cry. The families had recently been talking about a joint vacation, but there were no concrete plans yet. It all came to a head at that moment.

"Jay, I need you more than you know. I want us to travel together. I need you to do things with Lili and Andrew that I can't. Take them on hikes. Go for rides on jet skis. Play sports and games with them on the beach. I have become less active and more passive. They deserve to experience and enjoy the world and the unique adventures that every destination has to offer."

Within one week, they finalized plans to travel together. Three families with six children. On March 11, 2018, Lobio's 46th birthday, they left for Mexico.

"No matter what, just know that we are always here for you, for Christine, and the kids," Jay said.

He reassured Lobio. Even though Lobio had always felt that support, he needed to hear it. He needed his family and he was lucky to have them.

Being in Mexico offered a temporary escape from his personal burden. Not only was it a distraction from this disease but it was an escape for Christine, Lili, and Andrew. To enjoy the beauty of a tropical paradise with family, both nuclear and extended, was perfect. Lobio never did ride a jet ski but Lili and Andrew did with his brothers-in-law. Lobio watched and enjoyed that spectacle. He could not run full speed into the ocean like he used to, but this did not stop him from walking into the ocean and subsequently getting smashed by incoming waves with Andrew and his nephew, Jack, by his side. In fact, it was Jack that found Lobio's prescription sunglasses in the shallow ocean water with his foot. Lobio had been smashed by a massive wave, knocking his glasses off. When the white water cleared for a split second, Jack made the fortunate discovery. When Lobio was swimming, no one could tell he had any physical difficulties. His kids went on a couple of little excursions with the family while Lobio remained back, and this was okay with him. The kids were happy, excited, and safe. He was content watching them enjoy themselves. At some point during the trip, Christine told Lobio that her brother-in-law, Chris, made a comment to her: "Now I see." He was alluding to the noticeable changes in Lobio's walking pattern when increased distances were required.

Six weeks later Lobio travelled again, this time to California where he spent some time in San Diego in addition to a couple nights in the desert on the outskirts of Joshua Tree National Park. He experienced the daytime dry, scorching heat and evening briskness that only the desert could offer. The unique rugged landscape had a serene silence—interrupted only by the chatter of his family and friends, or music. Here the blackened night sky shone with distant stars, back home their twinkling diluted by the city's lights. On this trip, Lobio travelled with two of his brothers and a group of friends. His brother, Kevin, would be getting married the following month. While away, the group often did things at Lobio's pace. Having said that, if they wanted to go on excursions that he did not feel fit for him, he gave them his blessing.

Lobio ultimately concluded that he could still travel. The circumstances would be different and not what he anticipated but he could still see, smell, and feel the world. He and Christine resumed planning vacations. Foremost, he wanted his family to see Italy, the country where his parents were born. He hoped that as a family they would experience a gondola ride in Venice. He wanted them to be surrounded by saints within the surreal St. Peter's Basilica. He would always smile as he pictured them savouring gelato as they gazed over the beautiful city of Florence from the Piazzale Michelangelo. He wanted them to appreciate a wood-fired pizza in his father's hometown. He had seen these places and now desired his family to have the same memories. Lobio asked Christine if she was prepared to push him in a wheelchair if it came to that. Of course, she said yes.

Fatigue often stopped Lobio in his tracks. He learned that with MS, fatigue was characterized by a sudden loss of energy, such that the individual was not able to continue an activity that was physical, mental, or both. It was not the same as the tiredness or exhaustion that people without MS experienced. An individual with MS who experienced fatigue felt as though they were hitting a wall and could not concentrate. It is important to note that MS-fatigue cannot be worked through. When it strikes, it is "game over" for the time being. Recovery from this type of fatigue is prolonged.

Individuals with MS can experience two types of fatigue. Primary fatigue is the direct result of the disease process. In particular, the central nervous system needs to cope with areas that have been damaged by MS lesions, so an increase in energy expenditure is required. Secondary fatigue is a consequence of living with MS. Pain, sleep disturbances, medication side effects, depression, and stress contribute to secondary fatigue. Fatigue was an issue for up to 80 percent of those suffering from MS.

When fatigue would strike, Lobio was done and needed to get away. He needed to close his eyes, put his head down, and think about nothing. At times, he needed to do this for just a few minutes, sometimes fifteen to thirty minutes. This helped him considerably. Some need to lay down. Lobio knew the warning signs. His co-workers recognized it as a gaze: he would look straight through them, not absorbing anything they were saying. When this occurred, his co-workers encouraged him to step away for a short time as they would oversee the care of his clients. Similarly, his clients would also recognize the signs indicating when he needed to step away. After a short period of rest, he felt refreshed and he was back to himself. He was better able to do his job or any task at hand.

There were other ways that MS impacted Lobio's lifestyle. At different times in the past, he had thought:

"What should I have for dinner tonight? I feel like fast food."

"There is a *Star Wars* marathon on TV tonight. It carries on until two o'clock in the morning. Oh well. I only need a few hours of sleep. I should be fine tomorrow."

"Which pair of shoes should I wear to work today? I have so many to choose from. Comfort doesn't matter so much. It's about the colour and the style."

As the disease took hold of Lobio, he found himself accepting the inevitable and he eventually settled for a gradual decline. A significant amount of planning would go into his eventual choices. He would need to be both creative and shrewd with respect to planning and decision-making.

"There are factors that I am unable to control but there are many that I can."

The field of nutrition was dynamic and continued to evolve as both quantitative and qualitative research was committed to the subject. There had been extensive studies devoted to diet and the impact food can have on both health and disease. As related to MS, trying to identify the best diet possible could be mind-boggling. There was no "MS diet." Having said that, Lobio was consuming food that was predominantly plant-based, while including lean meats, healthy fats, and increased fiber. He was eating so much better and could honestly say that he felt better. He would never go as far as saying that his symptoms had reversed but he had realized the benefits of eating healthier: from feeling less bloated to having more energy. He also felt more mentally satisfied. And yes, there were some foods that seemed to make him drag his body more. He was still trying to establish a clear association, listening to the feedback that his body provided.

Supplementation with vitamins was also on his radar. Perhaps there was no more important vitamin for him than vitamin D. It was well-established that this vitamin was essential for bone health as it regulated the absorption of calcium. It had also been linked to a healthy immune system. There had been studies linking vitamin D deficiency to MS (Marin Collazo, 2020). There were sources of vitamin D in food but from what he understood, exposure to sunlight was the greatest source. Sunlight induces a chemical reaction in the epidermis of the skin, which ultimately results in the synthesis of vitamin D. Regarding medication, Lobio would require discipline to maintain compliance with his disease-modifying therapy as well as his daily oral pills. Disease-modifying medication could take the form of oral pills taken daily or injections taken a few times per week or infusions administered either monthly or spaced months apart. The selection of an appropriate medication was dependent on several factors including patient preference and the nature (aggression) of the disease. He understood that the disease-modifying medication might not mitigate his current symptoms but rather reduce the risk of future flare-ups. Lobio placed his faith in his treating physicians. With guidance from his neurologist, he elected to go with a medication that would be infused once every six months.

Regarding work, he would need to settle for a less lucrative, more manageable, and less taxing path. For this reason, he elected to leave the private sector where the caseload and pace were too much for him to handle. He returned to the public sector, working full time at the hospital where he began his career. It was the right decision to make and he had no regrets.

Lobio began to identify triggers that would temporarily flare his symptoms. In addition to working too many hours, he identified a lack of good sleep and a lack of rest throughout the day as culprits. If he was too tired, his day could be arduous. So, he would work and then come home and rest before dinner. He began going to bed earlier. In time, he would no longer need those rest periods before dinner. He attributed this to a good night's sleep and more manageable work habits.

Ironically, too much rest throughout the day would not serve him well. His legs would stiffen up to the point that when he needed to get up and walk, he would move like Frankenstein. As mentioned earlier, he would be stiff-legged but also ataxic. It was best for him to take short walks throughout the day. Sometimes at work he would stand while assessing clients instead of sitting for prolonged periods.

The importance of exercise could not be overstated—not just for Lobio, but for everyone. Exercise, in whatever form, came down to choice. There was always a way. He needed it not just for physical well-being but also for mental well-being. It was a necessity that he made time for.

Perhaps Lobio's biggest trigger was stress. Stress was an accelerant and could ignite the disease. Despite this being well-studied and documented, he did not need a textbook or journal article to tell him; his body conveyed this valuable yet unfortunate information. The effects could be lasting. Whether it was stressing about something insignificant like a pair of shoes that were not neatly put away at the front entrance or something significant like the illness of a family member, his body reacted adversely, with poor control of his extremities and ataxia.

"Like my mom said, I need to let things go." This was his mother's most powerful advice. Lobio knew he had conceded in many ways by letting many things go, but he still needed to continue down this path for the sake of his survival.

Lobio was continuously adapting to the ways that his new body worked. He was trying to survive the best way that he could with the biological makeup he had been given. He was listening. He was certainly not always happy about it. In fact, respecting his body's new needs was often monotonous, annoying, and frustrating, but he was listening. He was compelled to find a middle ground—a feasible balance between activity and rest. He had time and he wanted more.

Despite recognizing the relevance of a handicapped parking permit, Lobio struggled to give in to this label. In a way, he felt taking this step was giving in to the disease. It took him time, but he ultimately came to the realization that this would reinforce his own acceptance of the disease. He had not envisioned how much freedom this permit could offer him. He ceased isolating himself. Going out in public became more palatable. Previously, he was too worried about perception. He was not anymore. Lobio had feared going out into the world because he speculated that people were analyzing him from his head down rather than looking at his face and into his eyes. In fact, what came with acceptance was acknowledging that he needed help. His forearm crutch provided him with physical support, and if he aspired to be out, walking around in public with a crutch far exceeded staying home without a crutch. It took a long time to relinquish his independence of a gait aid, but when he finally did, he appreciated the freedom.

Lobio felt he was addressing his physical needs, but that he was neglecting his deeper-rooted spiritual needs. He drifted. God became distant. Lobio never blamed God for this cross that he carried but he became too obsessed with the biology of MS. Time wasted on prayer was simply getting in the way.

Eventually, Lobio appreciated that he could not believe in his body without believing in his soul. He was still chasing the biology of MS. It was what God would want him to do. Having said that, he was now devoting time to prayer and to the reflection on the person he was—to his essence, buried even deeper than the demyelinating plaques ravaging his central nervous system. Giving of himself, through teaching and especially through charity, would become a wonderful result of prayer.

"I have so much. Despite MS, I have good health. I am managing every minute of every day. Sometimes, I am pissed off and have had enough. But I have learned that tomorrow will begin anew. I can relate to others with disabilities. I believe I can help them. I pray that I can."

Lobio could argue that the healthcare professionals, especially the physicians, who directed his care knew so much more than he did about the pathophysiology of MS. However, he did know a little. And Lobio knew what MS felt like 100 percent more than them, assuming none of them had MS. He could feel what worked for him and what didn't.

One evening he was lounging in his backyard. The leaves from the surrounding trees rustled in the wind. It was dusk. Out of the corner of his eye, he spotted the tiny yet spectacular bioluminescent glow from a firefly. Thankfully the mosquitoes weren't biting. He was contemplative.

"What would it be like not to have MS? I've been there before. Life seemed relatively easy. Life was good.

What would it be like to have MS? I'm there now. So many simple tasks are so difficult. But you know what? Life is good.

I wonder how I can spin a chronic, unpredictable disease into something positive?"

Lobio hoped that people could learn from him. This was not arrogance. Rather, it reflected a surrender to the disease and an acknowledgement that transparency would boost him as he dealt with it. People were inherently curious, and many would ask questions. Lobio would tell them what he knew and what he didn't know. He would tell them what he felt. Teaching others was a way to teach himself. It was a way to feel he was contributing. He had the opportunity to teach physiotherapy students as they completed their clinical placements at the hospital. In later years, he had the opportunity to teach physiotherapy students at his alma mater, the university and school of physical therapy where he received his degree. He hoped the students left his lecture with a better understanding of MS and, more importantly, a better understanding of what it is like to live with a chronic disability. He even had the occasion to teach medical students. These second-year students were assigned to him to learn how to complete musculoskeletal assessments. However, he could no longer hide the fact that he had neurological signs and symptoms. These students were astute. Their curiosity was piqued. Their observational and analytical skills were developing. The result was a learning experience that rightfully tied both the musculoskeletal and neurological systems together.

Lobio had initiated in-services for his colleagues. Perhaps he could provide them with new ideas and tools as they treated others with MS. Lobio had become a resource for clients who were dealing with this disease and its ever-changing management. Family and friends were learning more about the disease than they would have ever imagined. It all came down to one important truth: Lobio could be a voice for those suffering from MS because he knew what it felt like to live with it.

Giving had always been so much more gratifying than receiving, at least for Lobio. Sadly, for a time MS had even taken that joy away from him. He found himself wanting more and more.

"I want to sleep through the night without waking up to take a piss . . . three times. I want to take a long, soothing, hot shower without feeling drunk afterwards. I want to kick the soccer ball around."

Why did he gravitate toward physiotherapy? Quite simply, it was because he felt most complete when he was helping and support-ing others.

Lobio made a conscious and purposeful decision to open himself up to the world. He would put his own vulnerability to good use. He would take advantage of it to help those who were more vulnerable than him.

When he thought of people linked to charity, the usual names came to mind: Mother Teresa of Calcutta. Bill Gates. Bono. There were so many others. These individuals were certainly inspirational. They had contributed to their respective causes and they had gal-vanized so many others to contribute as well. In some cases, they compromised their own well-being, safety, and reputation in favour of service to others.

What about Nikki Sixx. Who was this guy? Should his name be included on Lobio's list?

Nikki Sixx was a founding member of the heavy metal band Mötley Crüe, established in 1981. His excessive partying, drug use, and otherwise extreme lifestyle were chronicled in his book *The Heroin Diaries: A Year in the Life of a Shattered Rock Star.* The book was released in 2007. Lobio had always been fascinated by the lives of musicians; their biographies and autobiographies captivated him. And he loved Mötley Crüe. They peaked when he was in his teens. Lobio picked this book up to read stories about people who, in many ways, led lives on the opposite end of the spectrum to his. As he flipped from page to page, he could not believe what he was reading. He could not believe that Sixx was not dead, either by his own hands or someone else's. His life seemed like a perpetual train wreck. And for the most part, it seemed self-inflicted. Lobio felt duped. Here was a band and a rock star who were so creative and so influential on him in his youth, yet the more he read, the more he wished he had not been a fan. Yet, Lobio could not stop reading. Not because of the stories but because he needed to see if and how Sixx turned things around. He miraculously did. Not only did he save his own life, but he saved the lives of others by sharing his story of redemption. To this day, he contributes through his music, photography, writing, and charitable endeavours while remaining clean and sober.

Despite never being imprisoned by a drug or alcohol addiction, Lobio realized the Sixx's story was in some ways relatable. MS was what shackled Lobio. The key that freed him was his acceptance of the disease and his willingness to open himself up. Sixx wrote: "My heart's like an open book, for the whole world to read."

Lobio smiled. "I feel the same."

Lobio's work as a physiotherapist may be viewed by some as charity but he was getting paid to do it. He could give more and wanted to. Recently, Christine and Lobio formed a team for the local MS walk. This annual walk raises money for MS research, and to support those directly impacted by the disease. Lobio was proud that they had the biggest team and raised the most money. And this was just the start. Like teaching, charity offered Lobio a much-needed release. Having the ability to help others did his heart good.

Who's Helping Who?

†he door opened. Lobio gazed upon a world that he longed
to be in and one he did not want to be a part of. It was a
place he was meant to be in, but also one he wanted to run from.
He was torn. This paradoxical existence persisted as a tug-of-war
between Lobio and himself. Lobio sensed that he won and lost with
each pull of the rope. As he observed and evaluated those with MS,
he wondered if he would eventually experience the same struggles
with day-to-day tasks. He was overcome with a sense of melancholy.
Pondering his future, he became worried. As much as he knew that
the course of MS was variable, he could not help but anticipate the
worst. It was very difficult to distract himself from that thought as
he was often surrounded by the disease at work. He witnessed the
ravages of MS and other neurological conditions. There were times
that he simply did not want to be in the outpatient gym. As he
grieved, he chose to withdraw. When he was feeling this way, it was
best for him to get away. He would remove himself from the gym
after ensuring that his clients would be cared for by his co-workers.
On rare occasions, he would go home. Not only did Lobio need
to be away from the outpatient department, he needed to be away

from his profession, at least temporarily. If he was struggling to take care of himself, then he would certainly struggle to take care of his clients. He was grateful that he worked with a supportive and understanding team.

When Lobio was feeling completely indifferent and his mind was not on MS, this disease still hovered over him, like a dark cloud preparing to release a downpour. He was always striving to coexist better. He believed that he was. Acceptance from his clients helped him to ignore the disease and allowed him to better serve them. He hoped that he would continue to provide his clients with the quality physiotherapy they deserved. As time would go on, perhaps he would become more disabled. Perhaps not. His hope was that this dark cloud of self-pity surrounding him would progressively dissipate. Christine once remarked, "I hope you find your smile again."

"It's somewhere on my face. I guess it's hard to find; it's most often disguised by a frown."

On a workday, Lobio would enter the gym with purpose. He carried his files and water bottle in his left hand. His right hand firmly grasped his crutch. He looked toward his first destination: his co-workers were sitting at a table at the other end of the gym, preparing for the day. He hoped to arrive there without incident. Lobio concentrated. "Walk steady. Pick up your feet. Take your time. If you stumble, own it."

He was first obligated to pass by a couple clients or their supportive family members. "Good morning. How are you today?" Lobio inquired.

Generally, they would smile and reciprocate with, "Fine thanks, and, how are you?"

"I'm good thanks." For Lobio this little white lie was often the response he felt would best serve everyone in the gym.

Lobio walked on by and headed to his workstation. If he happened to have a good sleep that carried over into a good morning, his gait pattern was only mildly impaired. Nonetheless, it was noticeable. "I wonder what happened to him. Sprained ankle? Broken hip?" Lobio imagined people thinking.

Not only did Lobio sense their wonderment, they would often ask him, or they would ask his co-workers. He had advised his co-workers that if people did ask, he wanted them to know the truth. He had nothing to hide.

"Who is that guy with the crutch? I thought he was a patient but then I saw him sit down at your table with some files."

His co-workers would respond, "That's Lobio. He is a physiotherapist. He works with us."

"What happened to him?"

"He has MS," they would advise.

The response from each client had always been positive thereafter. Lobio knew this because his co-workers often reported these interactions to him. He hoped he was doing right by his colleagues by continuing to work with them. He wanted to be neither a distraction nor a source of comparison. Lobio had a job to do, but they did too.

Lobio's eyes were often fixed on the parallel bars as they were firmly planted around the perimeter of the gym. They were common pieces of equipment used by the physiotherapists to work specifically on balance. Strengthening exercises could also be incorporated. The goal of using the bars was to improve an individual's ability to stand and walk. From the outside of the parallel bars, a physiotherapist would provide instruction and direct an individual through an exercise routine. Was this where Lobio would be? On the outside? Or would he be on the inside receiving instruction? Seeing those parallel bars and pondering that very question frequently made him anxious. He could not foresee the future. No one could. But what he did know was that this was a chronic disease and it was generally progressive.

"I don't know if the parallel bars are there to help me or to mock me. Inner turmoil has overcome me. I don't think I can concentrate on my purpose right now."

Perhaps Lobio could exist both within and outside of the parallel bars. Or even better yet, maybe he could take advantage of these bars and use them to assist with his own physical rehabilitation as he worked with his clients. This was exactly what he decided to do. While prescribing exercises using the parallel bars to his clients, he would closely supervise them from within. He would demonstrate a specific exercise and subsequently perform the same exercise with his client. He would complete the same number of repetitions and with the same amplitude and duration. Occasionally, he would work on a completely different exercise while supervising his client with their exercise. This was a win-win situation. He had always been very physically active but now his new sport became a regimen of mundane balance, stability, and control exercises. Given his symptoms, these exercises were a challenge. In fact, they were not mundane at all.

Lobio often became solemn while at work. Attempting to deal with the physical losses that came with the condition was difficult, to say the least. Maintaining emotional stability while dealing with these losses could be impossible. It was not clear if his presence had a positive or negative influence on others dealing with MS or similar conditions. He did not know if he should be open or closed. Would his clients still feel comfortable working with him knowing that he was physically impaired? Could he remain objective in his role as their physiotherapist? Would the degree to which he exercised compassion change? Where did his co-workers fit in on this journey? As he mulled over these questions, he realized that the answers were not black and white.

Lobio deduced that it was best for him to remain open. He would always respect an individual's choice to be open or closed about their condition and even life in general. For him, being open had become a personal choice that came with no regrets, but it had presented some challenges. He had not been looking for sympathy or pity. What Lobio had decided to petition for most was understanding and acceptance. He wanted others to understand why he walked a certain way and why he often required the support of a crutch. He wanted them to understand why his hand shook when he was holding a pen and why he occasionally dropped things. He wanted them to understand why he needed to go to the washroom so frequently. Most importantly, he wanted them to understand that he was still very much alive, and he was the same Lobio on the inside.

For the most part, he liked to think he was putting a positive spin on this unique situation. All health conditions, as he came to understand, were unique. Even those with the same diagnosis experienced different symptoms and emotions. There were often objective findings and clinical signs that were consistent. Having said that, subjectivity was autonomous and Lobio had evolved to appreciate and respect this. No individual with MS experienced the same subjective and objective findings. But what he could do now was relate. As he was a physiotherapist, his best advice was to fight. This is what he had to do. He fought with every step that he took to get from point A to point B. He fought to steady his hand as he held a pen or eating utensil. He fought to keep his balance as he turned a corner as he walked. He fought for a restful sleep. What were his choices? There certainly were times that he just wanted to stay in bed and "get to it tomorrow," but then he would just be failing himself and those who needed him. And yes, there were still many who needed him.

Ironically, he often found himself defending MS. It was not well understood. He had been ignorant to how it presented until it impacted him directly. When people heard the diagnosis, "multiple sclerosis," they automatically visualized an individual who was or eventually would be bound to a wheelchair and was or would be completely dependent on others to function daily. This could be the case for some with MS but most often it was not. The comments and questions from clients often triggered sad emotions or daunting premonitions:

"My wife had MS and she died in a nursing home."

With a puzzled look, Lobio asked back sarcastically, "She died from MS?"

"You have MS and you are still walking?" another queried.

"I shouldn't be walking?" Lobio asked?

"It doesn't look like you have MS," she responded. Once again, Lobio asked, "What does MS look like?" She didn't know how to respond.

"Why are you still working?" asked a patient, as if MS was Lobio's golden ticket to a life "free", (at least that is how this man saw it), from (meaningful) labour.

"I shouldn't be working?"

"Lobio, are you going to be a vegetable?" Lobio was at a loss for words. "Wow. That's a new one," he thought.

Another was trying to make a joke. "You are going to be my physio? It looks like you need it more than me." Lobio continued with the assessment and held back from the response that he wanted to deliver: "I probably do."

Finally, his (least) favourite: "You don't know what it's like. One day, you might find out." Dejected, Lobio felt that he was finding out.

He was sure there was no malice intended with these comments, but they had planted seeds in him, nonetheless. It was clear that this condition was a mystery to many and often the worst possible scenario was what they envisioned. MS presented itself in many shapes and sizes. If those he encountered did not understand MS, then he owed it to the disease, and more importantly to those who suffered from it, to educate them. He was in a position where he could relate as both a healthcare provider and as a patient.

Lobio decided that he would remain open moving forward. He was not always like this. Dealing with his father's sudden and brief illness, impending death, and eventual death in 2005 shaped him in this way. That had been the most difficult experience of his life, until MS. Dealing with this disease ultimately became his greatest challenge. He still relied on his father for the strength to cope. One of the most effective coping mechanisms for him was to talk about it. It came easy to him to talk to those he was closest to. It was easy to talk to the medical professionals treating him. It was not easy talking to outsiders. It was most difficult talking to his clients. How and with whom he chose to discuss this took a great deal of thought. For a long time, he was able to disguise his MS. Now he could not. The physical signs were present for all to see. For Lobio, trying to keep his diagnosis a secret was a challenge he would lose. However, by being open, he believed this would enhance his battle against MS. This also served to garner acceptance and understanding from his clients.

"Why are you limping today?" asked Mr. Smith.

Rather than be completely blunt and advise Mr. Smith that he had MS, Lobio's response was a volley of questions back: "Am I? Why? What do you notice?"

Mr. Smith would often provide Lobio with detail. Lobio wanted to know, what Mr. Smith perceived from his viewpoint. Mr. Smith did not need a medical education to observe. Lobio was so appreciative of Mr. Smith's feedback. From his observations and analysis, Lobio was better able to decipher what it was he needed to work on. Lobio was helping Mr. Smith manage his respective physical condition but Mr. Smith was also helping Lobio deal with his. When all was said and done, he would tell Mr. Smith that he had MS and that he was grateful that he had provided Lobio with valuable information that he would use to his advantage. Another win-win situation. He would ask Mr. Smith if he had any questions. If so, Lobio would take the opportunity to tell him what he knew about the disease.

Despite being able to relate to others with MS, Lobio's personal story was different from theirs. Notwithstanding, he was still drawn to them. Lobio's co-workers, who had his best interest at heart, often tried to shelter him from clients with an MS diagnosis. It was often to no avail as Lobio could "sniff these individuals out." He surmised it was best that he knew who they were and saw how they functioned. He didn't want to make assumptions as he needed to see the truth and to deal with this reality. He, like them, had MS.

As Lobio continued to work in the outpatient department, he noticed that those with MS who knew he was dealing with the same condition were drawn to him. It was like a magnetic force of attraction that could not be disrupted. As much as he was watching every step they took, he realized that they were often evaluating Lobio's level of function as well. They often fed off each other. They bounced ideas off each other. Lobio felt that clients with MS who were better able to connect and relate to a healthcare professional that was enduring the same battles felt empowered to push themselves harder. The feeling was mutual; he had also received a great deal of support and encouragement from his clients who presented with other diagnoses. In some cases, they had told Lobio they pushed themselves because he pushed himself. He motivated them.

One day, Lobio was sitting at his workstation, his head buried in paperwork. A co-worker's client, the victim of a stroke, tapped him on the shoulder. As the man was tearing up, he said, "I want to thank you. You don't know what you have done for me. I have heard what you are dealing with and yet here you are, working hard, doing your job well and most importantly, smiling and encouraging those you are working with."

Lobio responded, "I want to thank you too. You don't know what you have done for me. It's people like you who motivate me to push myself."

It was moments like this that affirmed for Lobio that he was in the right place; "I have a purpose here."

No matter the diagnosis, they were all fighting battles together. They did not have complete physical control but one of the ingredients for improvement was the same for everyone: EXERCISE. This had been studied thoroughly and was well-documented in the literature. MS was not a choice. Exercise, tailored to a person's specific needs, was.

Being objective had always been a mandate of physiotherapy. Physiotherapists were driven by objective change. Measurable change most often dictated the need for ongoing formal physical rehabilitation. Without objective findings, it was difficult to discern if an individual required continuation of treatment.

Discerning when a client was ready for discharge from formal physiotherapy had always been one of the most difficult aspects of the profession. Objective change was the greatest benchmark, yet Lobio was firmly influenced by subjectivity. He had always had a soft spot for people, especially those who were dealing with a health crisis.

Due to his own health crisis, he had become more objective. He eventually dwelled on the disease less and less and was evolving as a physiotherapist. He was driven much more by objectivity and less by subjectivity. He would serve clients best by providing them with the tools to self-manage their respective conditions. He knew this because it was what he had to do for himself. There was no cure for MS. Lobio had complete trust in the medical professionals who were looking after him. However, most of the time he was away from them, essentially on his own. His doctors were not holding his hand and forcing him to lift weights, work on his balance, or go for a walk. He needed to be diligent and push himself. There was not a magic pill. Or was there? He believed that exercise was transformational. It was not a pill that would cure, but a strategy that would maintain his desired level of function. Physical rehabilitation was his profession and his doctrine. Lobio had grown as a physiotherapist and preached the importance of exercise to all his clients. He was sure that as he had gained clinical experience over the previous two decades, his analytical and practical skills had improved. Having said that, dealing with his condition had made him more objective than ever. If he had to engage in exercise to combat this disease, then so did they to combat theirs. Lobio would continue to provide encouragement, support, and the necessary tools but ultimately it was up to the clients.

Lobio took pride in the fact that he had always been a "go-to" physiotherapist. If there was a client that was known to be difficult, perhaps based on expectations or personality, his manager would say, "Give that new referral to Lobio. He has a way with difficult people."

Lobio was sure that not everyone would say that he could help them with their respective physical issues, but nonetheless he hoped that the vast majority of people he had the privilege of treating would say it had been a positive experience. He hoped they would say that he listened attentively and did not brush things off. He hoped they would say he made them smile and laugh, and if they needed to cry, he gave them a hug. Lobio always provided his best effort for his clients.

One of Lobio's co-workers approached him with an observation. She commented that as he worked with his clients, she would watch him interact with them. She said he was charming, and that she noticed his clients would always leave feeling better. At times, they were not necessarily feeling better with respect to their symptoms, but they were leaving their session with a smile. She told him he had a way of making a positive out of a negative situation.

Lobio recalled working part-time as a home care physiotherapist. He had received a referral to see an elderly widow who was living on her own. In her eighties, she had recently recovered from a medical condition that required a prolonged period of hospitalization. She was weak and deconditioned. Upon being discharged home, a referral was made for some home care physiotherapy. She required a regimen of strengthening and balance exercises. Her goal was to remain at home and continue to live independently. She and Lobio were permitted to work together for five to ten sessions. Upon completion of these sessions, the woman asked Lobio if he would continue to see her. He recognized that what she wanted more than anything was companionship. So Lobio visited her once a week, no longer in his capacity as a physiotherapist, but as a friend. She would always have a fresh batch of homemade cookies and a tall, refreshing glass of orange juice ready for him. As they shared the cookies, they would discuss a TV show they both enjoyed. Sometimes she would provide an analysis of the book she was reading. Later, they would stroll up and down her street with her arm entwined around his. She would tell him about the neighbours living in each home, sometimes telling him too much. She reminisced about life on her street. Sometimes they walked together in silence. They walked on beautiful days. They walked when it was raining. They walked through the snow. Lobio knew she looked forward to these visits and so did he. She became a close friend. She even befriended Lobio's wife and soon afterwards, his infant daughter. She had since passed away but had been an integral part of his life. Lobio was referred to her because she required physiotherapy. He wanted to remain in her life because she became one of his friends. She was there for him then and he knew that she would be there for him now, were she still alive. He had continued to visit her regularly because it was the right thing to do, but more importantly, because he had wanted to.

Despite his own hardship, Lobio sensed he could never lose his compassion. Before he was a physiotherapist, he was a compassionate person, finding people of all walks of life to be fascinating. This was one of the reasons he was drawn to his profession. Since being diagnosed with MS, he found that he could empathize more with his clients, but he would not sympathize. He still felt for the clients he treated, supporting them emotionally within a reasonable capacity, but he would also push them within their tolerable limits. He would not let them quit. If Lobio could snap his fingers and make MS go away, he would. There would be no hesitation, but he simply could not do this. One of the ways he had accepted his illness was by using it as a tool while he engaged in the physical rehabilitation of others. He had gained some control by making this situation mutually beneficial. He was placed in a unique position, forced to deal with MS, initially from the outside and subsequently from the inside. He was his clients' physiotherapist but because of an implausible reality, they too became his.

Aside from Lobio's immediate family and a couple of his closest friends, there had been no others more on this journey with him than his co-workers. In fact, he could argue that they had been involved the most. They became his family away from home. He developed a dependency on them that extended beyond needing physical support. He needed them emotionally.

When his initial MRI pointed to MS, Lobio was glum as he pondered his future. He was able to hold it together for his clients. But he was not the same person. He became withdrawn. His co-workers were there to cheer him up and to encourage him. They arranged for a social outing and they treated him as if everything about him remained unchanged. Lobio reciprocated. He needed these nights out. At the end of one evening he was in conversation with one of his co-workers. He said, "I don't know where this is going but I hope I can remain at work."

She responded. "Please don't go. You make this place fun."

Lobio smiled.

His co-workers were driven by the same thing he was: the need to help others. Now, he needed help. He was both co-worker and client to his colleagues. They would continually aid Lobio. Eventually, it became second nature. The flow of treatment continued for his clients because his co-workers were there for him.

As time went on and the disease took hold, Lobio had decided that when an opportunity arose, he would return to the hospital full time while cutting back at the clinic. In the summer of 2016, there was an opening at the hospital. A new position was established but it did not seem like a good fit for Lobio. However, if another co-worker filled that position, their vacant position would become available. One of his closest co-workers filled the position, which opened his up for Lobio. The colleague felt his position could be a good fit for Lobio, and he knew what Lobio was dealing with. He took a chance and made a big sacrifice in leaving the comfort of a position he had held for so many years. Lobio applied for and accepted the resulting opening, which incorporated work in Outpatient Rehab as well as Pulmonary Rehab. Lobio's colleague always maintained that he had been looking for a change. Maybe he was but no matter what he said, Lobio felt that his co-worker did this for him.

Lobio did not want to be a burden on his co-workers. He didn't want them to work harder than they already did. This disease was for him to deal with, but they were indirectly affected. He always felt this diagnosis tested him and would continue to do so in ways that continued to surprise him. However, this diagnosis would test his colleagues too. They were helping him to manage a difficult situation. Most importantly, to them he was still Lobio.

It Only Takes a Smile

As devastating as the disease was, it hurt Lobio more that the people that he cared about the most were forced to witness what was happening to him. They would say things like, "I don't know what to do. I wish there was more I could do. I don't know how to act when I am around you."

Lobio often didn't know how to respond, other than saying, "I'm sorry that I make you feel this way." But he understood. Those that he was closest to, whether it be family, friends, or co-worker, had a relationship with MS that was intimate yet indirect. Lobio frequently felt it would serve him best to look at himself through other people's eyes, as he might understand and cope better. To them, "M" and "S" were just two letters of the alphabet.

As Christine's husband, Lobio appreciated that no role in his life had been more neglected than this one since his diagnosis. He felt like a failure.

"Christine, you can do a lot better than me. 'For better or for worse'. You had the 'better.' I guess now you get the 'worse.'"

It wasn't just the MS, but the emotions and the moods that it carried with it. Lobio thought, "It's not fair to her. Would it be better for her if I was gone and she could carry on with life? I would be a memory. In many respects, I am already just a memory."

The reality was that there was no individual who had shared this diagnosis with Lobio more than Christine. She was the one constant. She enabled Lobio to see the light at the end of the tunnel. When he was down and wanted to be left alone, she left him alone. She did not pry or push. She didn't interrogate him. She knew. If he wanted to vent or talk, she was there. She held him when he clearly needed to be held. Lobio could not dance with her but he could listen to music with her. He could not go for a run with her, but he could watch her run. They could watch together as the kids competed in their respective sports. He could mope all the time and expect her to take it. Or he could joke and laugh, just like he used to, and know that at that very moment she felt, "he's back." Lobio tried every day to see the fun in life. He saw those good things in her face. When he arrived home from work and he knew she would be there, he felt relief and happiness, even if it did not show on his face. It was there . . . always.

"When I stare into your eyes and you are looking back at me, this disease is all but forgotten. As I lay in bed next to you and gently place my hand in the crook of your arm, I feel the spasticity in my legs subside. I'm not sure that you know what power you have."

When Mother's Day came around recently, Lobio presented her with a card. In it, he wrote one sentence: "Without you I would be in a gutter."

That summed it up.

Lili and Andrew were survivors in their own ways. They were neither from Christine nor Lobio, but they were theirs nonetheless, and vice versa. The disease had changed Lobio's role from the "run and play with us at the park" papa to the "let's walk to the park and you can keep an eye on us as we play" papa. He was less active and more passive. The kids understood that if some form of physicality was required, Lobio was not the person to go to. They had several uncles, aunts, and cousins that not only loved them dearly, but enjoyed spending time with them. These relatives were all more than physically capable of joining Lili and Andrew in play. This had been difficult for Lobio to accept. Angry outbursts for reasons other than his own resentment were once commonplace. As he had evolved and acceptance had permeated his persona, his kids had gravitated toward him. They knew what Lobio had to offer: unconditional love, support, and protection. He and Christine were their primary educators. They were learning the way of the world as Christine and Lobio saw it, and the parents were directing the children to reliable sources for answers they did not know. While coexisting with Lobio as they witnessed the sequelae of MS, the kids had matured in ways that not many at their respective ages had. Respect, acceptance, and support of those in need of assistance had permeated their youthful personas as well. Lobio was so proud of them. They didn't need to see someone with an assistive device to remind them that person needed help. They could recognize it in a person's face or demeanour. They had learned to be patient and compassionate. Lobio and Christine's children knew that people came in all shapes, sizes, and colours. They understood Lobio's limitations. More importantly, they respected them. Lobio knew that the day could come when he might need to get around in a wheelchair and he was sure they would be there to push him.

Lobio was driving home one afternoon with Andrew sitting in the backseat. They engaged in some deep conversation. Andrew clearly had some things on his mind. "Papa, if people are sick and they don't take their medicine they can die right?"

"It depends on why they need the medicine. What's on your mind?"

"If someone is sick with germs, they need their medicine."

"Yes, they do. Anything else?"

"If you have MS and you don't take your medicine, you will die."

"Whoa. Is that what you think? MS will not kill me. Even if I do not take medication. MS can make my life more difficult, but it will not kill me. I do not want you to ever feel that way. Okay?"

"Okay papa. I believe you."

Lobio would always be an educator to his kids. MS was just one topic of many. As much as he was teaching them, they were always teaching him. It would always be this way. Lobio had been self-absorbed for too long. He knew and felt his kids were bigger than him. Lili and Andrew would always inspire Lobio to feel better for them. Both children were living with a father facing a chronic and potentially disabling condition. They were taking it in stride. On Father's Day, Lili presented Lobio with a card that contained a beautiful note she had written herself. A small excerpt from this note states, ". . . We don't know what is going to happen in the future, but we can get through it together."

"How are you today?", Lobio's mother reluctantly inquired. Reluctant because she knew what Lobio's response would be and not because she didn't care.

He responded, "Breathing."

It was one of those days when Lobio woke up and was disappointed that he did in fact wake up. No matter how old he was, he always felt that he was his mother's baby. He initially tried to hide his feelings from her. This did not serve either of them. If he hid his feelings, he could not confide in his mother when he needed to. She could not help him if she did not know what was wrong. She was left feeling nothing but helpless.

Eventually he decided that he would tell her everything. She was learning about MS as he was. She was learning about Lobio. Both she and Lobio felt more at ease by discussing the truth. He felt so much better talking to her and he needed her hugs.

Despite his father's passing in 2005, Lobio's father remained an integral part of Lobio's life. He would continue to learn from him. When he was confronted by a big decision, he would ask himself, "What would papa do?" That is certainly not to say that his father was always right. There were times when Lobio felt his father had made the wrong decision, so Lobio chose a different path. His father's eternal presence had even strengthened Lobio's decision-making as he dealt with MS.

"I'm not sure how my father would have handled watching the way this disease has taken me down. He would have cried. But then he would have grabbed my arm and told me to 'toughen up.'"

On a balmy Sunday morning in June 2015, Lobio picked his brother up at their mother's home. They had a soccer game. "Mom just told me you got your MRI results. What does that mean? What will happen to you?"

"I'm not sure. For now, things are as they were. You don't notice anything do you?"

"Maybe you are a little slower playing soccer. That's it. We all are anyways."

"Yeah, I think that's it too. There are a few other little things, but you wouldn't notice these."

That's how it was back in those days. The MS was not noticeable to the outside world, Lobio's brothers included. They had witnessed Lobio's physical devolution and emotional hardship since the beginning. All that he could do was to be himself as best he could. They knew Lobio as their big brother. He could only imagine that it was tough for them to see him this way. They often felt helpless. Having said that, he did not feel helpless, knowing he had them in his life. If he needed something done around the house, they were there. They were always there for Lobio's kids and his wife. The best he could do was offer his brothers honesty. He was confident they would take it from there.

There was always an element of surprise and concern when a family member learned of another family member's change in health. Typically, this revelation was disclosed second-hand. "What? MS? I know someone with MS, and you would never even know it. He works full time, plays sports, and he seems to be in great shape."

Or the contrary. "What? MS? I know someone with MS, and he's in a wheelchair. He hasn't worked in years. His family does everything for him. He doesn't seem to do much for himself."

Whether it was an aunt, uncle, cousin, grandparent, niece, nephew, or in-law, the response was most often one of grief and worry. Any emotion that followed was dependent on the relationship with the individual who had been newly diagnosed. Since being diagnosed with MS, Lobio had learned ("felt" was a better word) who he could rely on. He had physical and emotional needs. Being an open person, he would remain cautious about the information he shared. Curiosity was simply that. However, he had some genuinely supportive family members, some of whom were blood-related and some who were not, who he could count on as he campaigned against MS. They, like his immediate family, enlivened him in ways that he was driven to open up. He was able to express himself truthfully. They wouldn't have to guess how he was feeling by the look on his face. He felt so comfortable with them that he was able to verbalize his feelings. He hoped this sharing was therapeutic for both parties. Lobio knew it was for him.

"I have so many friends. Actually, do I have any friends?" Lobio had been cogitative. How could a question like this even cross his mind? It came down to how he defined "friend." Was that person simply an acquaintance who he would say hi to in passing, or was that person someone who he was able to be transparent and vulnerable with? How would that person adapt to Lobio, "the guy I know so much about, who has this disability? How will Lobio continue to remain in my life? Likewise, how will I modify my own life and adapt to him?"

For Lobio, it came down to a feeling deep within. "How much will I let them in?"

Lobio often pondered his friends, especially those who were truly by his side during his journey with MS. There were people who provided him with constant unconditional support. He once told his mother: "I know it is impossible for you not to worry about me, but I want you to know I am surrounded by great people."

Lobio appreciated that this gave her great comfort. His closest friend, Jonathan, was a physician working and residing in another city. Coincidentally, Jonathan often practiced at the same hospital that Lobio's neurologist devoted hours. He even resided in that city. Having him by Lobio's side along the way was something that Lobio had never taken for granted.

"Lobio, I wish there was more I could do," Jonathan once declared.

Jon had done so much for him. He was a medical resource and provided Lobio with a place to stay when he was in the city for his medical appointments; it was far more than Lobio could have ever asked for. But most importantly, Jon remained his closest friend. He was his brother. He had introduced Lobio to a wonderful world of eclectic food, fresh ingredients, and wine. Lobio's taste and demands for good food became expensive. There were things in life, Lobio realized, that were often underrated and underappreciated. Savouring food, sipping wine, and socializing with close friends were a few of those things, best when they occurred all together. The simple pleasures in life! He had that with Jon. These were activities that Lobio could partake in, whether he was sitting or standing. They both loved soccer too, often shared vibrant stories. Lobio had known Jon nearly all his life—they grew up next door to each other. Firing off bottle rockets, ball hockey on the street, a misfired hockey ball launched by Scottie "The Winder," striking Jon's front door with his mother subsequently answering the ghostly knock, tobogganing down the local hill, and causing mischief with the neighbours were some of the experiences they had shared. Later when Lobio and Jon got together, they reminisced. The two men had countless chuckles, followed by more glorious wine. Minutes and hours would pass by. Moonlight would transform into sunrise; there would be little time left for sleep.

Lobio recalled staying with Jon and his family for about a week while he was undergoing treatment. Lobio saw how well Jon's clothing fit. Somewhat fashion conscious, Lobio often found it difficult to find clothes that fit him well as he had a slender frame. So did Jon but with greater height.

"I will take you where I buy my clothes," Jon declared.

"That would be great!" replied Lobio.

Lobio assumed it would not be cheap, and he was right. As soon as he tried on a button-down shirt at this establishment, he was not going to leave without it. The colour was outstanding. The fit was perfect. Upon returning home, one of the first things he did was sort his laundry for cleaning. Christine noticed the shirt.

"That's a nice shirt. Is it new? I haven't seen it before."

Lobio told her that it was in fact new.

"When did you get it?"

He advised her that after spending a week away from his family and undergoing treatment, he had wanted to treat himself. He went shopping with Jon.

Her response, "Oh no. We don't live on a doctor's salary. How much did it cost? $100?"

"Higher."

"What? For a button-down shirt? $150."

"Higher."

This went on and on until they reached the final price: $270. There were a lot of four-letter words exchanged. The lecture went in one ear and out the other; the shirt looked great on Lobio and he put it to good use.

Then there was Lobio's friend Ryan. Ryan was a successful physiotherapist who now ran his own practice. Lobio met him in the undergraduate biology program at the university. Lobio graduated with a bachelor's degree in science (biology) while Ryan stayed one more year to complete an honours degree. He followed Lobio to physiotherapy school a year later. Ryan was gifted at his trade. Lobio had always felt that if his mother ever needed physiotherapy, he would want her to see Ryan. To say that he was an excellent, intelligent physiotherapist was an understatement. He had been with Lobio all along. It was at his clinic that Lobio had to cut down his hours and eventually take a leave from. Lobio had missed working with one of his best friends. He missed the time they would spend together when all the clients had left, and they remained and chatted. Lobio was not sure there had been anyone he had been able to be more transparent with. He got the sense that Ryan felt the same.

Coincidentally, Ryan too loved soccer! In fact, it was Ryan that invited Lobio to join his local soccer team over twenty-five years ago. On that team, Lobio played at a competitive level for nearly twenty years. Most of the time he played on the same team as Ryan. However, on occasion they were opponents. Lobio remembered one of the later games. Afterwards, Ryan commented to his wife: "Did you see that?"

"Of course, I did," she stated. "You guys had a good game and you won."

"I know but that's not what I'm talking about. Did you see me get by Lobio on that one play?"

Lobio smirked as he thought about that moment. "What a flattering compliment. Savour this moment Ryan. I will be more prepared the next time."

Ryan too was like a brother. Lobio still had the keys to the clinic and visited regularly during off-hours to exercise. Ryan understood firsthand how important exercise was to him and his survival. Ryan's mother, too, had MS and had been fighting this terrible disease a lot longer than Lobio. Lobio cherished alone-time at the clinic. It was a time for him to focus on himself. He would spend a couple hours on balancing exercise and self-reflection while listening to a varied array of music.

Despite the admirable people in his life, there was a stretch of time that Lobio was in a state of despondency. Christine was able to locate a close friend of Lobio's through social media. He and Lobio had lost touch for no other reason than geography. They attended physical therapy school together. He had since become a doctor and was living and working in the United States. Lobio and Jens reconnected.

"Lobio! Long time no talk! How are you? Are you still playing soccer?"

As simple as the answer to that question would seem, Lobio did not know if their first contact in years should contain full disclosure. He decided that it should as he did not want to dance around the truth. Lobio told him. There was silence.

"I don't know what to say."

"There is nothing to say Jens. This has encompassed my life in recent times. Too much time, for that matter. I am doing okay though. I am managing. I am surrounded by many great people."

They soon discovered they both enjoyed riding their bicycles. However, it was becoming more difficult for Lobio to ride outside due to his balance issues and self-imposed safety concerns. Unbeknownst to him, Jens initiated communication with Christine about indoor riding. He took it upon himself to purchase the bicycle trainer and had it shipped to Lobio's house. This invaluable piece of equipment enabled Lobio to safely ride his bike, and through a popular cycling app, ride through various parts of the world, sometimes with Jens virtually by his side. Even though they lived over 2,000 kilometers from each other, they were able to ride together. The physical improvement in Lobio's health could be measured. The emotional benefit could not. The greatest benefit was that Lobio had reconnected with a friend who he had always shared so much in common with.

As Lobio was learning to coexist with MS directly, his friends were learning how to deal with it indirectly, provided that Lobio would let them in. There were several people within his circle who he knew cared a great deal about him. His life had run smoother because of it. They supported him at work. They included him in social outings. They continued to hug him.

Lobio knew that having a friend with a disability would be a challenge. Friends might say, "It would be easier if he just said he was not going out with us tonight." Or the contrary: "Let's choose a place that works for Lobio."

Some of his friends just got it. Lobio used to expect that his friends should get it. This was selfish of him and would lead to negative emotions and worsening physical symptoms. The disease had a sinister way of blending the emotional and physical together, almost instantly.

No one owed Lobio anything. However, in their own way, his closest friends gave him everything. It had taken him time to realize this.

"I have so many friends."

MS was a condition that Lobio's co-workers learned about a long time ago in school. Eventually, they were exposed to it on a regular basis as they assessed and treated clients with this disease. Little did they know, a co-worker would one day also become one of their clients. They would analyze Lobio's movement and provide him with advice on ways to manage and ameliorate his symptoms. Paramount to this, they were there to support him in any way possible as he provided for his clients.

There was a time when Lobio tried to hide his emotions from his colleagues. He believed he was protecting them, but in fact this approach led to more unease. They were apprehensive about asking him how he was doing. Lobio eventually realized that it served them all better if he was honest and accepted their offers of assistance. His co-workers had become indispensable as he coped with MS.

Lobio mused: "I am always watching. I will always learn from you. You are all my lifeline away from home."

Lobio thought about all his clients. "I am glad you have MS. Well not that you have this disease. You know what I mean. I'm sorry for saying that. It's just that you get it," disclosed one client to Lobio as a tear sprouted in the corner of his eye.

"You don't have to apologize. I understand what you meant," Lobio replied.

"What did I do wrong?" (with a vulgar yet understandable four-letter word inserted)

"Nothing. It's not your fault. It's no one's fault. This is life. I hear you. You are not alone. Neither am I."

Clients had a deep-rooted need to convey frustration and disappointment. Lobio was not equipped to help them to deal with their emotions, but because he was able to relate, they were often comfortable venting to him. Lobio was okay with this. This esoteric relationship carried with it a symbiosis that even propelled Lobio. When he gazed at these individuals as they were fighting various neurological disorders, they often had one thing in common. They were all smiling! These smiles had provided him with perspective and a positive outlook. This motivated him. Both Lobio and these "patients" could share in defeat and loss. They could encourage each other's efforts and celebrate their triumphs.

Lobio's employers were always supportive and understanding. He was employed within a department and facility where he would expect understanding. His superiors backed him right from the beginning. They had been accommodative and worked with Lobio to establish realistic working parameters. He knew that by him being transparent, they were more likely to be supportive. By being open about his condition, he had garnered endorsement from his managers and employers. He realized that he needed and wanted them on his side if he was going to effectively battle this disease.

What about those who shared the same diagnosis? "We MSers know what it's like."

Lobio had never heard this term before. In fact, the more that he thought about it, he did not want to be labelled as an "MSer." An individual with the same diagnosis enlightened him about this label. As time passed, he recognized that they shared much in common. Despite a difference regarding the physical manifestation, the emotional impact was often akin. This analogous relationship provided an opportunity to benefit both parties. He learned that connecting with the MSers offered an avenue to vent and, more importantly, to problem solve. Additionally, everyone had an interesting fact or pointer that they were able to bring to the table. Lobio remained careful as he analyzed all the information that was presented to him, but he felt that it was all valuable. "I am Lobio and I am an MSer."

How would strangers act around him? When Lobio would meet someone for the first time, he often wondered what their first impression of him was. First impressions and image held value for so many. A shaky hand or the use of a crutch could be perceived as a sign of weakness. Feeling that others were watching and analyzing him was likely one of the reasons that Lobio was often inclined to stay at home. In the end, he realized that he was making too many assumptions.

Lobio felt encouraged that so many individuals, whether they knew him or not, wanted to help. The perception of his mobility issues led to offerings of assistance. The people helping didn't need to know why Lobio was struggling with his mobility but if they asked, Lobio would tell them. He was often offered the opportunity to educate others regarding MS and this was not exclusive to his family or friends.

His spirituality and beliefs were certainly put to the test. Ideally, everyone had the freedom to choose their paths in life. The greatest gift that they had been rewarded with was free will. Everyone was special in their own way and everyone could contribute. Lobio also had faith in something or someone bigger. Call Him "God." Call it "science." To Lobio, it was both. This is what comforted him.

His conviction was that everyone was dealt the cards they were, and it was not a higher power that decided what these cards would be. Everyone had the free will to do with these cards whatever they chose. Lobio did not want MS. It was not God's fault that he had MS. He held dear to his heart that however he dealt with this disease and whatever choices he made, good or bad, a belief in Someone or Something that was bigger than him provided him with both inner peace and a sense of invigoration.

A Musical Companion

There was a song for every moment. Lobio's feelings were often reinforced by the music he was listening to. Except for the meaningful people that surrounded him, music was certainly his greatest ally.

As he sat back and reflected on his journey both with and without MS, he would envision how he arrived at every destination and immediately there would be a song that would accompany him. When he was a young adult and full of dreams, the song "A Silent Moment" by Elephant Stone from the 2013 album *Elephant Stone*, popped into his head. The possibilities were limitless.

Upon graduation from physical therapy school, he gained successful employment, got married, bought a home, started a family, and lived life to the fullest. "Summer of '69" by Bryan Adams from the 1984 album *Reckless* captured the happiest times of his life.

Upon being diagnosed with MS, Lobio soon hit the lowest point of his life. He envisioned a bleak future, one filled with progressive decline and misery. He felt that "happy" was no longer a word in his vocabulary. He would listen to darker music. One song that was so powerful and difficult to escape was "Fade to Black" by Metallica from the 1984 album *Ride the Lightning*. Lobio felt there was nothing left to give. Life no longer made sense to him. The end did.

With a heavy heart and some deep reflection, he accepted that he was mortal and broken. The song "Fragile" by Sting from the 1987 album *... Nothing Like the Sun* and "Moment of Surrender" by U2 from the 2009 album *No Line on the Horizon* supported him. He needed to step away from work for a period. Only by accepting his own vulnerability would he be able to capture his identity and embark on a new journey. The song "Freewill" by Rush from the 1980 album *Permanent Waves* reminded him of his individuality and bolstered his desire to find purpose. When he listened to the song "Just Breathe" by Pearl Jam from the 2009 album *Backspacer*, he would smile as he thought about what he did have and not what he didn't.

As Lobio made a conscious effort to better himself physically, mentally, and emotionally, the song "Coming Back to Life" by Pink Floyd from the 1994 album *The Division Bell* sustained him. As he reflected on the people who were vital to his perpetual battle with MS, the people that he loved so dearly, the song "In Your Eyes" by Peter Gabriel from the 1986 album *So* would bring him to tears. This song was appropriately his wedding song.

When Lobio returned to work, he was worried that he would be seen and treated differently. Perhaps people would expect less of him. "Don't You (Forget About Me)" by Simple Minds from the 1985 album *Once Upon a Time; Deluxe Edition Disc 2; B-sides and Rarities* asserted that both his co-workers and his clients viewed him as the same person he always was. Their expectations remained unchanged.

Lobio eventually recognized that he had the fortitude to live with MS. The song "In the Light" by Led Zeppelin from the 1975 album *Physical Graffiti* affirmed that everyone was in search of light and that it would always prevail over darkness.

Looking ahead, perhaps there was no more fitting song than "Let Down" by Radiohead from the 1997 album *OK Computer*. Despite being interpreted in many ways, this song made Lobio hopeful for the future. He knew that he would have to abide by certain parameters. Despite a sense that all was lost, there was a glimmer of hope that would propel him to unexpected heights and places.

The songs that Lobio listened to at any given moment would release a much-needed emotion. They might place him in the moment and fortify the notion that he was not the sole person dealing with a seemingly insurmountable obstacle. They might take him out of the moment, offering an escape from the same obstacle.

Lobio knew that no matter what would transpire with his health and no matter who would come and go, music would always be there for him. Its presence could literally be heard wherever and whenever he wanted and, imperatively, when he needed. He was not alone.

A New Adversary

During the early months of 2020 a disastrous menace engulfed the globe: COVID-19. This challenged everyone as the scourge of the virus spread virtually unchecked.

Lobio was faced with a new dilemma.

"Should I stay home and patiently wait it out while hiding from this unwelcome invader or should I go to work and potentially expose myself? My immune system is compromised. If I do become infected will I be able to fight it off? Most importantly, what is in the best interest of my family?"

To establish a reasonable solution, Lobio needed to consider his emotions and his physical needs. Based on previous experience, he knew that a lengthy time away from work brought him down with respect to both needs. Without work, he would no longer need to awaken early. Despite the desire to remain active, he would not be compelled to get up and move throughout the day. His walking abilities would suffer. He would minimize human contact with both those who were able and notably those who were disabled, the latter with whom he shared a common bond. He would distance himself from the analytical thought process that was required of him every day as a physiotherapist.

Lobio decided that it was essential for him to work. This would serve his family best by helping him to remain as functional as possible. Amid the chaos that was COVID-19, he wanted Christine and the kids to see normalcy in him. His employers, who had all been ceaselessly supportive, decided for him that he would not be involved with direct patient care. He would remain in the outpatient department, essentially working by himself, completing phone checkups with clients as well as through the evolving telehealth system. This was the best-case scenario as he would be able to exercise both his mind and his body.

The pandemic aside, Lobio realized that the lack of activity, both physical and mental, exacerbated this disease. The risk of separating himself from these vital needs far exceeded the risk of going to work during a time of crisis, such as COVID-19. He would remain ever vigilant.

"MS makes me feel like crap, so I am going to push myself even harder. I am going to work. I am going to ride my bike. If not, I lose."

Lobio also came to the realization that home was not a house. His own house, with Christine, Lili, and Andrew, was where he felt most comfortable. It also felt like home when he was sitting on the couch next to his mother as they discussed world events. Sometimes he felt at home when he was in a lotus position, surrounded by silence and laden with a sense of melancholy, within a few feet of his father's headstone. Sometimes, he felt at home when he was at church, listening attentively to Father Mike's homily. Sometimes, he felt at home when he was in his brother's backyard pool, wading with a draft beer, all the while watching a soccer game on the big screen. Home was a place in his heart, and it was a sense of identity. MS was not just about not being able to walk. It was about not being able to be. For his heart to beat most efficiently, Lobio needed to exist in more places than his house. This was moulding him into the purposeful person he wanted to be.

Adapting to a New Environment

What was the definition of "alive?"

"Alert. Animated. Active. Not dead."

These were a handful of interpretations of alive. Lobio was aware of many individuals who were not active, yet they remained very much alive. He was also aware of many people who were awake and yet they seemed dead. His own interpretation of alive had evolved. If not, he would continue to plummet deeper into an abyss.

Previously, Lobio's interpretation of the word alive revolved around the word "routine." There were activities that were essential: eating, sleeping, bathing, grooming, working . . . repeat. There were milestones that could be used to measure quality of life: finding a mate, getting married, having children. There were leisure activities to fill the time in between and these activities offered great satisfaction . . . hopefully. For Lobio, some of these were playing soccer, listening to music, watching sports, watching movies, travelling, socializing, and doodling. Of course, there was valuable time spent with family and friends. The list of things to spend time on went on and on and was unique to everyone.

Undoubtedly, MS was never the best thing that ever happened to Lobio. Not even close. It was the worst. However, it had certainly provided him with a new perspective, and it had caused him to discover new ways to survive. For far too long, hope was lost. Negative emotions, such as fear, took over.

"Fear can hold you prisoner. Hope can set you free."

This moving quote was taken from *Different Seasons* which was a collection of four novellas written by Stephen King in 1982. The 1994 film, *The Shawshank Redemption,* directed by Frank Darabont, was an adaptation from one of these novellas, *Rita Hayworth and Shawshank Redemption.* For so many years, his eyes would often gaze upon a poster in his basement of that movie bearing that quote. It was still mounted to the wall. This quote reminded him what he needed to do but he eventually came to the realization that it was not just about doing. It was about feeling. Buried deep within his heart, he felt hope.

He hoped that one day there would be a cure. More, he hoped that those much brighter than him would prevail in their efforts to regrow myelin, so that damage could be reversed. He hoped that science would continue to make leaps and bounds with the goal of eradicating this disease. He hoped that the physicians and health-care professionals who were looking after him continued to have his best interest at heart. He believed and felt that they did.

He hoped that his family and those he was closest to would continue to tolerate him.

He hoped for him. He hoped that he would be able to free himself from the unremitting grasp of MS. He hoped for the fortitude, and most importantly, the will to persevere in his perpetual fight.

He hoped that he would have solid, uninterrupted sleep that evening because he was tired. He was looking forward to waking up the following morning!

With or without MS, he wanted to be the person he was meant to be, right or wrong, serious or funny, happy or sad.

TOMORROW

A Glow Illuminates
a New Path

Did anyone really know what the future held? Six years prior, Lobio felt invincible. He was doing everything right to reinforce both physical and mental fortitude. Aside from a transient visual disturbance and some other minor symptoms, he was playing soccer competitively a couple times per week, working in multiple settings, eating whatever he wanted, and sleeping as much or as little as he needed to. He was in better physical shape than even ten years prior.

"This will continue."

January 2016. Enter multiple sclerosis.
"No big deal. Life goes on."

One year later.
"Heat is really bothering me. Soccer is on hold for now."

One and a half years later.

"Ok. I concede. This is more than an inconvenience. I am hanging up my soccer boots. I'm sticking to my bike. I can't run anymore. I hope that there won't be a zombie apocalypse because I will certainly be their first feast. In only a couple years I have regressed from being one of the fastest guys to one of the slowest. I just want to walk. At least I am still working, and in both of the places that I want to."

Lobio was blinded by his temerity. MS, after all, was a big deal.

Two years later.

"This is the worst year I have ever lived. This is fucking bullshit. It's torture sometimes going to work and seeing clients with MS, all the while living with this same unrelenting disease. In addition to seeing it, it feels like I'm living my own horror day after day. I'm dragging myself. I am using my arms to carry my body. My legs, especially the right one, are failing. I need a crutch. Now I am embraced by this "MS hug" thing: burning surrounds my trunk and apparently "embraces" me to the point that I want no one to hug me. I experience numbness in my feet, lower legs, right hand, and to a lesser extent my left hand. The sensation that I perceive is, in fact, a lack of sensation. At least I can look forward to some sleep. No, wait. Even that is a nightmare even before I can fall asleep and dream a nightmare. My right leg twitches. Numbness has transformed to neuropathic burning throughout my feet, lower legs, and right hand. All this torments me as I am trying to fall asleep. When I do finally fall asleep, soon afterwards a sense of urgency will wake me. I better get to the toilet fast, or I will piss myself. Now, there is absolutely no time in a twenty-four-hour period that this disease will relent. I'm fading. I'm done. I need to get away from work. I'm going home for a while, maybe for good. To say that this disease is terrible is an understatement. When will it end? How will it end? I don't know."

Three years later.

"I'm going back to work. My co-workers are going to see me with a crutch. So will the clients I serve. Oh well. I can't sit around at home all day by myself and stare at the ceiling. It needs to be painted anyways. It looks like shit (frown)."

Four and a half years later.

"Going back to work was the best thing that I could have done. I'm stronger. I can lift my right leg without my hands assisting. I can bend my knees better against gravity. I'm not catching my right foot as I walk. Sometimes I walk without my crutch. I might look drunk, but I can still walk. People, for the most part, are so supportive. My clients are amazing. We work together. They push me as I push them. I need them. I am riding my bike indoors like crazy. My thighs are so muscular. They were not like this even when I was playing so much soccer. I never use my crutch now when I am home. It waits for me, resting next to the umbrellas by the front door. It is leaving marks on the front entrance wall. Now, this wall needs to be painted too. It looks like shit (smile). I still have so many symptoms, but I am acclimating to my ever-changing body. It is not just a downward spiral. I experience upswings too. I am hopeful. I am mentally stronger."

A Thought-Provoking
Change of Plans

Lobio realized that he could learn from the past, mould the present, and shape the future, all along knowing that his present condition would force parameters on both him and his family. As this journey unfolded, Lobio had learned so much about himself. Perhaps many of his negative emotions and insecurities predated his diagnosis, becoming amplified on that day in January 2016. What he believed would be just a little bump had turned out to be a rugged, jagged mountain with a peak that was often out of sight, obscured by dark, ominous clouds.

Lobio continued to learn, adapt, and evolve. He had never been a firm believer in fate, destiny, or "things happening for a reason" but he respected those who did. The way he saw it, life happened, and it was how people dealt with challenges that could make or break them. This disease had weakened him physically and may continue to do so. In conjunction with the physical deterioration, it had waged psychological warfare. This would present as an enduring battle. However, Lobio had never felt so mentally strong. Gaining mental strength had facilitated regaining physical strength. He was prepared for his new reality.

Lobio would have been overconfident and naive to believe that he would no longer experience bad days. He had been down that path before and he had fallen flat on his face. As a result, he was more prepared than before, and had the motivation to persevere. Lobio realized that the same darkness that speckled his brain in the form of demyelinating plaques was surrounded by light that wanted to break through. He had been holding it back.

"The cure is not yet attainable but the potential to ameliorate many of my symptoms is within reach."

The dark speckles were not under his control. The light was. For Lobio, the capacity to mitigate his symptoms had never been solely about a medication, a diet, a move to a more favourable climate, or an exercise. It was, perhaps, all of those. However, most importantly it was a choice. He had been thrust into a living arrangement whereby he was forced to cohabitate with a vexatious roommate who would simply not move out. He could choose to make the most of this arrangement or he could roll over in bed and fade away. The disease would press on.

Lobio's perspective of the world around him had changed in a positive way. Pessimism had shifted to optimism. Sadness was eclipsed by happiness. He had always been drawn to people and the need to make a difference. He found himself on the receiving end and graciously embraced it.

"Perspective. Should I lose my temper and scold Andrew for not making his bed or should I thank and hug him for sweeping the floor, for helping me to cut vegetables and prepare dinner, or for carrying a cup upstairs for me? The latter is so much more gratifying. Should I feel slighted just because my co-workers did not give me a pat on the back for a job well done or should I focus on how often they support me so that my job becomes that much easier? I choose the latter. Should I look through the window with frustration at the rainfall when I was led to believe that it was going to be a beautiful clear day or should I proceed outside with my arms raised and gaze upward, embracing Mother Nature's grandeur, all the while getting drenched? I am now inclined to choose the latter."

The crutch that Lobio relied on to support him when he walked had been a source of visual conflict. It had reminded him of dependence, frustration, and struggle. In the 2000 Robert Zemeckis film *Cast Away*, the stranded and lonely lead character, Chuck, portrayed by Tom Hanks, befriends, and ultimately loves a volleyball that he names "Wilson." Lobio's crutch had become his "Wilson." It often rested at the bedside and waited for Lobio. Sometimes he rested on the back seat of Lobio's car as he waited. Lobio was often walking within his home without his crutch, but it would always be close by. Waiting. Lobio would see him and feel settled. He felt comfort and at the same time, he felt bolstered. "I am here for you Lobio."

There could come a day when Lobio would no longer need him. There could come a day when Lobio might need to move on to another gait aid. Lobio would cross that bridge when he got there. Until then, his crutch was there for him. He reminded others as well that he was there for Lobio and that Lobio needed some assistance, patience, and time. He pointed out that Lobio was not invincible, vanity was superficial, and had no place in Lobio's life. This was an invaluable reminder to him. Perhaps his crutch deserved a name.

Lobio became most inspired by the human spirit. Yes, he was surrounded by loving family, friends, co-workers, medical professionals, and others who were consistently watching over him, but it was not them alone. It was the frail elderly woman who saw him with a crutch and insisted that he enter the store ahead of her. It was the early morning rumble of a lawnmower that Lobio realized was being pushed by his teenage next-door neighbour as he was grooming Lobio's yard without being asked to do so. It was the middle-aged male who recently underwent a painful knee procedure and divulged that he had no business complaining as he considered

Lobio's situation. It was the motorist who was clearly short on time but allowed Lobio to cut in front while in a line of traffic. It was Lobio's co-worker who had become a close friend and ally. He told Lobio that he recently learned some hands-on therapeutic techniques with an emphasis on neurological rehabilitation and he insisted on trying them on Lobio.

"Here's what I offer. Twelve sessions and my charge . . . free. All I need and expect from you is that you show up and work with me."

It was Lobio's children, who were neither conceived nor born to Christine and him. They began their precious lives halfway across the world. He still marveled at the fact that they embraced all aspects of life while living under Lobio's roof. "They are survivors." They inspired Lobio to push on.

"Who am I?" Lobio thought.

"I am Lobio. I am a husband. I am a papa. I am a son. I am a cousin. I am a nephew. I am an uncle. I am a son-in-law. I am a brother-in-law. I am a friend. I am a co-worker. I bleed Italian blood. I am honoured and privileged to call myself Canadian. I am proud to call myself a physiotherapist. I have been told by many that I am funny and quick-witted. I do have a dry sense of humour. At the other end of the spectrum I am also intense and deep. I am very sensitive and wear my emotions on my sleeve. I have a vivid memory for detail, like my father before me and my mother now. My favourite colour is blue. It brings out my eyes. I would like to think I have a keen sense of fashion. I strive to look my best. I love sports, especially soccer. I am inspired by so many genres of music. I enjoy a good drama, action, or sci-fi movie. A classic comedy can always brighten my mood. Reading captures my undivided attention. I crave knowledge. I love numbers. Math is sexy. Science provides captivating insight into the world and universe, and I am always curious. I played the alto saxophone for nearly one decade of my adolescent life. I can read music. I always love the sound of music playing in the background. I have always had a knack for drawing. Languages are fascinating and

I always try to pick up foreign words as I deliver physiotherapy. I have a good memory for those spoken words. Time spent creating in the kitchen is fulfilling. I salivate over the aroma of a succulent rack of lamb or the site of a beautifully plated dish of sushi-grade tuna. I have a sweet tooth and especially love cheesecake. If I never taste or even see a raisin again, I will consider it a great success. In fact, if someone told me that raisins were the cure for MS, I would still have MS. I take pleasure in a delectable glass of dry red wine, or a sip of whisky. I enjoy travelling and experiencing the world around me. The landscape. The people. The culture. I could rest comfortably on a beach and gaze out at the ocean for hours, simply taking in the sights, sounds, and smells. I am in awe of the natural world, especially the animal kingdom. If I was a species other than human, I would narrow it down to a dolphin, a killer whale, or a bald eagle. I feel humbled, cleansed, and rejuvenated when I go to church. I love, admire, and have a soft spot for people. Everyone has something to offer. Everyone has an engaging personal narrative to recount. This is just a little bit about me. Oh wait, there is one more tiny piece of insight . . . I move a little slower and sometimes seem awkward and clumsy . . . because I live with multiple sclerosis."

Embracing Life

Lobio woke up from a peaceful sleep and his day started anew. He sat up on the edge of the bed. "How will today play out? I slept well. The sun is shining. I feel it is going to be a good day."

Before starting his morning routine, Lobio gazed through the window, deep in thought. He reflected on the past. In particular, he recalled a somber day in January 2016, when he was diagnosed with MS. This was one of the saddest days of his life. Or was it? Only minutes before this unavoidable pronouncement, his youngest brother sent him a text and a photo. He and his wife had just welcomed their first child into the world, a bouncing boy named Gabriel. In the end, this day turned out to be one of the greatest days of Lobio's life. Gabriel exudes everything right and joyous about life!

"Perspective. Is the glass half empty or is it half full?"

The glass, Lobio decided, was both half empty and half full. His most recent sip contained MS and he would say that it had left a sour taste in his mouth and on his palate. He anticipated that the half remaining, which still was imbued with MS, would be rich in both bouquet and flavour. He would savour every drop and take his time doing so.

He wanted to hate MS, but he needed to love it. It was buried deep within him and would not be going anywhere. Lobio reluctantly, yet peacefully, embraced his fellow traveler. It was the only way to move on. Even with a loss of function, he had more to give. He had knowledge.

"I committed no crime, yet I permitted MS to imprison me for far too long. I will not tolerate this bondage anymore. I will remain assiduous as I plan. I know you will always be travelling with me, but you will sit your ass in the back seat."

He smiled, arose, and started his morning routine. Upon completion, it was time to leave for work. As it was so pleasing outside, Lobio elected to ride his electric trike. It was genuinely pleasurable. Beyond that, he was free again, outside, feeling the breeze brush by his skin as he safely raced down the trail on his way to work.

"There's always a way!"

As Lobio was zipping down the parkway on his e-trike, someone passed by him on his road bike. He looked back as he passed by Lobio and commented, "That's why you are going so fast. You're cheating."

Lobio grinned and thought to himself, "In your eyes I am cheating but in mine I am living."

When he was nearly at work a light drizzle came down. He finally arrived and the clouds split open. It was raining harder. He got off his trike, but he was not able to run into the hospital quickly. He would ultimately surrender to the inevitable. "I am going to get wet. That's all there is to it."

Careful and vigilant. It was preferable that Lobio would be wet and upright versus soaked and on the ground.

"Oh well. Such is life." Again, Lobio grinned. He was overcome with a rush of happiness. For the first time in a long time, he could not wait for what lay ahead.

"Hey Christine, guess what? I am finding my smile again!"

Epilogue

I am Robert. I am Rob. I am Robbie. I am Cusi.
I am Lobio. My father called me by this name. It had neither a meaning nor a translation. It was simply an affectionate nickname.

This story is a series of snapshots of my life since being accepted to physical therapy school and receiving my MS diagnosis.

New York Times bestselling author Richard M. Cohen also has MS. In his book *Chasing Hope: A Patient's Deep Dive into Stem Cells, Faith, and the Future,* he wrote: "I kept reminding myself that I am more than my illness. Who I am is in my head and heart, in my soul, not in my sneakers." There could be no more fitting words to depict my current plight. It has taken time and experience to come to the same epiphany.

As physiotherapists learning the craft, we are instructed that objective change is paramount in measuring progress. But what about subjectivity? Does it matter if someone has full range of motion and strength in his knee, yet experiences so much pain that he never leaves the house, instead electing to lead a sedentary life? By contrast, his neighbour can hardly bend his knee, yet he enjoys eighteen holes of golf a couple times per week. Does it matter if someone appears to be in fantastic physical shape yet feels he cannot join his friends downtown at a pub because he is embarrassed that his bladder will let him down? Conversely, one of his friends is very out of shape and appears older than his chronological age, yet he will be there, relishing the experience with no worries other than the bill at the end of the night.

I have learned through my battle with MS that I am only as good as I feel, not as I do. And by "feeling," I mean mentally. Many of the symptoms I experience are here to stay. Sometimes they are manageable and sometimes they are not. This disease will be buried deep inside me until I take my last breath. Until that time, I must cope. Not only because I need to but because I want to. I want to make the most of my life. Mostly I want to be the person that I was before MS.

People use a variety of coping mechanisms to deal with life's challenges. Food, sports, friends, reading, and movies are some that come to mind. Self-destructive choices such as drug and alcohol dependency also come to mind. I have no shortage of trustworthy coping methods. Riding my bike, cooking, enjoying food, and quality family time are right up there. But music is always there in the background. Sometimes it pushes itself to the forefront and there it flexes, all by itself. For me, there is no stronger influence than music. Music is ceaseless, with new talent emulating past talent, or creating their own unique genres. I have a deep relationship with this art form. When a melody accompanied by lyrics enters my ear, is processed, and is electrically transported to my temporal lobe, it does not just sit there. It then shoots off to my frontal lobe and other regions of my brain. Finally, the electrical impulse fires off to my heart. The result is that what I hear feeds an emotional need. The most influential poets in my life are, in fact, lyricists. Their message once again remains crystal clear: I am not alone.

I tell my kids:

"Hey Lili, I would love for you to play me a song on the piano. You are creating beautiful music and I hope that you appreciate your talent."

"Hey Andrew, I want you to pound those drums. I love listening to you! You, too, are so talented."

The symphony that I hear within my ears encourages me to tolerate the sensations throughout the rest of my body and encourages me to take that one extra step, whether it is walking further or painfully fighting for that one extra sit up. I am relaxing in the living room, all alone. Words simply do not do justice to the beauty visible outside. It is early May, one of those cloudless days where all you can see are blue skies that extend to eternity. The temperature could not be more perfect. The birds are singing. There are squirrels everywhere, scavenging the neighbourhood. Even the sound of a lawnmower humming in the distance is music to my ears. My nose catches a whiff of a recently mowed lawn. I just came in from outside after a few hours biking with Andrew. Well, he rode his bike while I sat on a park bench and timed him riding various routes. Ironically, today was supposed to be the annual MS walk. It was cancelled this year due to the COVID pandemic. I elect to play one of my father's records. I inherited these when he passed away. I dig up "A Touch of Tabasco," by Rosemary Clooney and Perez Prado. My eyes close and I am transported to another place. I am at the home that I grew up in. I walk from the kitchen into the dining room as I am heading out to look for my father. He walks into the dining room from the patio door. We meet. We are separated by a couple feet and facing each other at a standstill. The sunlight from the window behind me shines brightly into his face. His eyes are a brilliant aqua blue just like they always were. He is once again wearing an oversized baseball cap as well as a beaten-up pair of glasses. He is holding his cup of coffee with another cigarette in his mouth. His other hand is empty. He is not holding an envelope this time. He reaches out to me and places his calloused hand gently on the side of my face. I lean my crutch on the dining room table. Just like always, it slides along the edge, falls, and comes crashing down to the floor. Except, this time I don't hear the thump. Cuban music is playing in the background. He comes in closer. His smile is warm and comforting.

"Lobio."

"Yes Papa."

"I'm proud of you. You can do this . . . Tough."

He would randomly say that word to my brothers and me. "Tough." He would clench his fist and make an uppercut toward the heavens. We knew what he meant: "The world is tough. Life can be tough. You be tough right back."

And with that, he places his coffee cup on the dining room table and tosses his cigarette butt into it. He comes in closer. He wraps his arms around me. I return the hug and rest my head on his shoulder. He, like so many others, is my crutch. I don't need my own forearm crutch right now. I cry.

My eyes open and I am once again lounging comfortably on my chair in the living room. Cuban music still serenades me. I am crying because I need to. My tear-filled eyes are also a brilliant aqua blue, just like his were. The smell of coffee, grappa, and smoke is gone. The hug is not. I feel his embrace. I stand up. Like always, my legs shake for a few seconds and then it fades away. I reach for my crutch. This rather simple, yet ingenious assistive device reminds me that there will always be a way. I breathe deeply. Then I take a step. And I live.

And I'm free.

References

1. Doidge, Norman. 2007. *The Brain That Changes Itself*. New York (US); Toronto (Canada). Penguin Books.

2. Marin Collazo, Iris. 2020. "Vitamin D and MS: Is there any connection?" https://www.mayoclinic.org/diseases-conditions/multiple-sclerosis/expert-answers/vitamin-d-and-ms/faq-20058258

About the Author

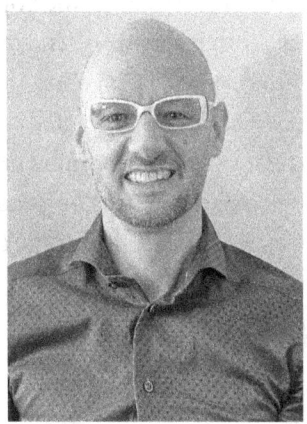

Robert Cusinato is a physiotherapist born, raised, and working in Windsor, Ontario, Canada. He graduated from the University of Windsor with a Bachelor of Science (Biology) in 1994. He then went on to graduate from Western University (formerly the University of Western in London, Ontario) with a Bachelor of Science (Physical Therapy) in 1997.

His career has embodied work in the public and private sectors, homecare, and long-term care. He has also had the privilege of teaching physical therapy students at his alma mater, Western University and medical students studying at the Schulich School of Medicine and Dentistry, Western University.

Over the years, he has worked with individuals of all ages and with varying diagnoses. He has garnered a genuine interest in multiple sclerosis over time, especially while working in the outpatient neurological rehabilitation department at a local hospital. He has been inspired by the battle that he has witnessed every day when he is at work. Victims of aggressive diseases with relentless symptoms provide their greatest efforts to survive and live a life despite knowing that they may always be bound down by physical impairments. Given the prevalence of MS in Canada, he and his family have been involved in charitable causes for the last five years in support of those dealing with this disease and in the hope that one day there will be a cure. He has written this story as a testament to all those battling chronic disease that despite all odds, there is always a way.

Outside of work, he has always gravitated towards an active lifestyle with a keen interest in soccer and more recently bicycling. He also has an eclectic taste in music that bolsters him with everyday activities. He is appreciative of the gifts that he has been given. He is an enamored husband and proud father of two.

CPSIA information can be obtained
at www.ICGtesting.com
Printed in the USA
BVHW050352190822
644900BV00001B/27
9 781039 100008